The Elements of Managed Care: A Guide for Helping Professionals

Susan R. Davis
Private Practice
Linwood Psychotherapy Services

Scott T. Meier
State University of New York at Buffalo

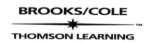

BROOKS/COLE

™

THOMSON LEARNING

Australia • Canada • Mexico • Singapore • Spain
United Kingdom • United States

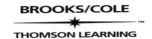

BROOKS/COLE
THOMSON LEARNING

Counseling Editor: Julie Martinez
Editorial Assistant: Marin Plank
Marketing Manager: Caroline Concilla
Signing Representative: Tricia Caruso
Project Editor: Matt Stevens, Teri Hyde
Print Buyer: April Reynolds

Permissions Editor: Bob Kauser
Production Service: Shepherd, Incorporated
Copy Editor: Francine Banwarth
Cover Designer: Ross Carron
Compositor: Shepherd Incorporated
Printer: Webcom, Ltd.

Printed in Canada
1 2 3 4 5 6 7 04 03 02 01 00

For permission to use material from this text,
contact us by
Web: http://www.thomsonrights.com
Fax: 1-800-730-2215
Phone: 1-800-730-2214

Wadsworth/Thomson Learning
10 Davis Drive
Belmont, CA 94002-3098
USA

For more information about our products, contact us:
Thomson Learning Academic Resource Center
1-800-423-0563
http://www.wadsworth.com

International Headquarters
Thomson Learning
International Division
290 Harbor Drive, 2nd Floor
Stamford, CT 06902-7477
USA

UK/Europe/Middle East/South Africa
Thomson Learning
Berkshire House
168-173 High Holborn
London WC1V 7AA
United Kingdom

Asia
Thomson Learning
60 Albert Street, #15-01
Albert Complex
Singapore 189969

Canada
Nelson Thomson Learning
1120 Birchmount Road
Toronto, Ontario M1K 5G4
Canada

Library of Congress Cataloging-in-Publication Data

Davis, Susan R., 1956–
    Elements of managed care : a counselor's guide / Scott T. Meier.
        p.   cm.
    Includes index.
    ISBN 0-534-54974-8
    1. Mental health counseling—Practice—United States. 2. Managed mental health
care—United States. I. Meier, Scott T., 1955– II. Title.

RC466.D38 2001
362.2'04256'068—dc21   00-43371

ISBN: 0-534-54974-8

Table of Contents

3   Managed Care and the Counseling Process   35

Preface

We believe that managed care has emerged in the 1990s as the single most important influence on the practice of counseling and psychotherapy. The impact has been most strongly felt by full-time practitioners who must deal with managed care on a daily basis, and it is this group that has been the intended audience for almost all books published on managed care. In contrast, few books have appeared intended explicitly for students and beginning professionals.

Administrators of counseling agencies have told us that graduates are unprepared for dealing with managed care. One administrator and clinician described new counselors as "not having a clue" about managed care. Because managed care has become a central agent in determining the form and content of mental health delivery in nearly all settings, faculty and clinical instructors increasingly recognize this area as critical to students' future success. Consequently, more graduate programs are beginning to include managed care as a major or special topic in practica courses and professional seminars. Nevertheless, any course which deals didactically or experientially with the practice of counseling, psychotherapy, diagnosis, and assessment would be an appropriate place to introduce students to issues surrounding managed care.

Thus, the major goals we have for this book are to provide (a) an introduction to major issues related to managed care and counseling and (b) an impetus for discussion and increased awareness of these and related issues in graduate students. Because many faculty do not function as full-time clinicians, they have not experienced the sometimes overwhelming impact of managed care on mental health services and counselors. Consequently, this book should provide an important bridge that will enable instructors to convey a sense of the important problems and clinical experiences in this domain to students who will soon be attempting to cope with managed care. Our presentation of scholarly and applied information about managed care, coupled with multiple real-life examples of managed care's impact on clients, counselors, and the counseling process, will provide students with the needed breadth and depth of knowledge necessary to begin to practice and cope in this environment.

We have long-term optimism about prospects for the counseling professions and short-term concern about the effects of managed care. Ample evidence exists documenting the need for and general efficacy of counseling (Bergin & Garfield, 1994). Despite this, managed care has blanketed counselors and clients with a host of restrictions, designed to hold down costs, that have adversely affected the quality of available and provided services. One result is that the overwhelming majority of mental health professionals and health care professionals in general hold negative opinions about managed care (see Committee for the Advancement of Professional Practice, 1995; Miller, 1995, 1996). Health care professionals frequently refer to "mangled care" or "managed cost care," and the general public increasingly shares these negative perceptions.

From the perspective of many counseling and mental health professionals, the current state of managed care has relatively few redeeming features. Managed care *has* succeeded in reducing rapid increases in health care costs, although some think this is only a temporary state (Sauber, 1997a). Similarly, one reviewer of this book related an instance in which the arrival of managed care in a rural area motivated mental health agencies to improve their counselors' credentials from bachelor's level to certified or master's degree. Managed care companies, however, often appear out of touch with values held by the counseling and the health care communities. Originally designed to emphasize prevention to maintain health (Roberts, 1998), HMOs' top priority now appears to be short-term cost-containment and profit, with quality of care often a distant priority.

After 10 years of direct experience with managed care companies, along with a fairly extensive knowledge of the literature, we see the outcomes produced by these companies as often more harmful than beneficial. From an ethical and moral basis, we cannot simply recommend that counselors be "managed care friendly." That had been the attitude recommended by many educators, authors, and experts in the early and mid-1990s who then believed that managed care was a necessary, albeit overwhelming force that the helping professions should adapt to for our sake and our clients' welfare. But as we document in this book, in many instances managed care companies have demonstrated little concern about the welfare of clients or counselors. Managed care companies have typically reduced costs not through increased efficiency, but by simply reducing mental health services to clients and cutting funding to service providers. We cannot in good conscience recommend more of the same.

This book's format is similar to that of the *Elements of Counseling* (Meier & Davis, 2000): a combination of theoretical and empirical knowledge, supported by multiple practical examples, briefly presented. While distilling the key elements of counseling is not easy, accomplishing the same task with managed care is even more complicated. Managed care procedures vary across companies and regions over periods as short as a few months. What remains the same about managed care, however, is its underlying philosophy. From the perspective of practicing counselors, managed care's emphasis on short-term cost and profit, to the detriment of quality of care, often produces common issues for counseling and mental health professionals across companies, settings, and occasions.

Those common issues are the focus of this book. First, we believe it is important for counselors to understand the historical development of managed care. Chapter 1 begins with a description of the economic and governmental factors that facilitated managed care's recent growth; the second part of this chapter then lists a number of the problems managed care has subsequently created or failed to address. The parameters imposed on counseling—that is, the explicit and implicit rules of managed care companies—are discussed in Chapter 2. Chapter 3 focuses on how managed care has changed what transpires between client and counselor during the counseling interaction. Chapters 2 and 3 provide a first-person perspective by presenting many actual examples of counselors' and clients' interactions with managed care companies. Problems and possible improvements in outcome assessment, a potentially important method for feedback and monitoring of quality used by managed care companies, are discussed in Chapter 4. Finally, Chapter 5 describes a range of approaches with the potential to improve managed care practices and related health care problems. A major goal of this chapter is to encourage students, counselors, and faculty to consider professional, scientific, political, and social action related to managed care.

Because managed care has introduced an entirely new language to the counseling professions, a Glossary and an Appendix are included at the end of the book. The Glossary contains key terms organized alphabetically, while the Appendix presents those terms arranged thematically. Readers who have no managed care background may wish to begin with either the Appendix or Glossary before proceeding to the main chapters. And given the speed with which the debate about managed care changes, counselors will need to keep abreast of these discussions through professional and popular sources. We hope to facilitate this process by providing a list of useful Internet sites in Chapter 5, all of which are accessible through the second author's homepage (www.acsu.buffalo.edu/~stmeier/).

Our primary thanks are to the practicing counselors, clinicians, therapists, and counselor trainees who shared their managed care knowledge and experiences with us. We also acknowledge the helpful assistance, comments, and suggestions of four graduate assistants, Benson Hendricks-Hoffman, Elizabeth Letsch, Elizabeth McGough, and Jennifer Sapia; the book's reviewers William H. Blau, Copper Mountain College; William Buffum, Barry University; James David Cross, Houston Community College; Tim Davidson, University of Oklahoma; John Liptak, Wilmington College; Joan Polansky, Lewis & Clark College; and John Rigney, Lindsey Wilson College; the production editor Matt Stevens; and the Editors, Julie Martinez and Eileen Murphy.

Finally, we should note that both authors contributed equally to the writing of this book and that the order of authors is alphabetical.

Susan R. Davis, Ph.D.
Scott T. Meier, Ph.D.
January 2000

The Causes and Consequences of Managed Care

In the past decade the helping professions have been turned upside down. While costs were always a concern—few agencies, for example, could ever boast of having more staff than they needed—the methods of managed care have placed systematic and substantial constraints on counselors in agencies, schools, hospitals, and private practice. A multitude of methods have been employed to control costs, including limiting the number of sessions, restricting who may provide services, delaying payment for services by weeks and months, and continually pressing for or imposing lower fees (Kessler, 1998; Rabasca, 1999). Brief therapy is now the norm in most settings; some clients may be eligible for only two to three sessions annually (Shore, 1996).

How did the helping professions move from a focus on delivering the best care to a struggle to provide basic services? This chapter provides an answer by reviewing the factors that led to the rise of managed care.

Cost increases in health care

The most frequently cited reason for the ascendance of managed care is that government and business have searched for decades for ways to restrain health care costs. Cummings (1996) maintained that during the 1980s "mental health costs skyrocketed and became one of the most significant contributors to the health care inflation spiral" (p. 213). Mordock (1996) estimated that medical costs were rising at twice the rate of inflation and mental health costs at twice that rate. Goodman, Brown, and Deitz (1992; also see Davis, 1998) cited Gray (1991) as reporting that health care expenditures rose from 6 percent of domestic spending in 1965 to 12 percent in 1992 and are expected to be about 15 percent when this book is published. Goodman et al. (1992) also cited data indicating that while 3 percent of the population uses psychiatric insurance benefits, psychiatric treatment accounted for 25 percent of all hospital days in 1987 and 30 percent in 1988. Some observers suggest that the United States spends more on health care than any other nation, but with no better outcomes and coverage of a smaller proportion of the population (e.g., Newman & Reed, 1996).

In the United States most people receive their health care through employer-provided medical plans; the United States is the last advanced industrial nation which does not provide national health insurance (Andrews, 1995). One of the reasons for managed care's ascendance is that managers of American corporations began to notice the magnitude of health care cost increases: in 1984, for example, health care costs equaled one-third of corporations' pretax profits (Califano, 1986, cited in Broskowski, 1994). By 1997, 85 percent of employees in employment-based health plans belonged to managed care insurance plans (Pedulla & Rocke, 1999).

Why did costs increase?

Who or what is responsible for these rising costs? Among the factors that have been listed as contributing to general health care cost increases (Broskowski, 1994; Davis, 1998) are:

- an aging population who use more services,
- rising expectations for health care (i.e., people expect health care to be available),
- more medical malpractice suits,
- a disproportionate amount spent on administration of the health care system by managed care organizations (estimated at 24 percent by the Robert Wood Johnson Foundation, Center for Health Economics Research, 1993), and
- improved medical technology.

In the arena of counseling and psychotherapy, however, Cummings and Sayama (1995) laid the blame at clinicians' feet. They indicated that before managed care, the mental health practitioner effectively made all cost decisions:

It is the doctor who decides what is to be done, how and when it will be done, and in the case of psychotherapy, how long it will take. . . . As intrusive and arbitrary as managed care can be, when the practitioners had the control there was no incentive within their ranks to reduce costs by increasing efficiency and effectiveness. (p. 29)

Similarly, others claim that "mental health costs were the fastest rising costs throughout the 1980s" (Patterson & Sharfstein, 1992, cited in Corcoran & Vandiver, 1996, p. 23).

Too much inpatient care?

The idea that all mental health costs have been spiraling out-of-control turns out to be an oversimplification. Scholars have noted that "costs for *outpatient* mental health care were not increasing at the same high rate as other forms of health care, and . . . outpatient mental health care is only a small piece of the overall cost of health care in the United States" (Welfel, 1998, p. 321; Iglehart, 1996; italics added). Similarly, Broskowski (1994), an insurance company representative, wrote that "professional psychologists have not been primarily responsible for creating the cost trends that have stimulated managed care in mental health" (p. 1). While general medical costs increased between 12 percent and 20 percent between 1959 and 1979, mental health costs increased only 3.5 percent over that period (Kiesler, Cummings, & VandenBos, 1979).

Newman and Reed (1996) argue that during the 1960–1990 period, health care policy emphasized acute care, surgery, and short-term general hospital care and de-emphasized outpatient procedures. Newman and Reed (1996) believe that "providers have actually had economic disincentives to emphasize prevention, early intervention, and treatment in less restrictive environments, and in general, to mount serious initiatives to maintain health, as opposed to providing medical interventions focused on existing symptoms or illness" (p. 14).

Our analysis of the literature is that for-profit hospitals and the executives who ran them have been largely responsible for mental health cost increases. While the government or charitable/religious organizations primarily owned hospitals prior to the 1970s, in that decade for-profit hospitals "became a big industry with potential profits, and it attracted many investors and entrepreneurs" (Broskowski, 1994, p. 8). Where have these profit-oriented folks focused? Although only 10 to 20 percent of all users need inpatient care, 65 percent to 80 percent of alcohol, drug abuse, and mental health (ADM) costs occur in inpatient and residential settings (Broskowski, 1994). Broskowski (1994) reported that in 1990 a 28-day inpatient stay for alcohol or drug treatment cost around $15,000. Other observers have reached similar conclusions:

> The vast proportion of mental health care costs are incurred through the use of inpatient services. (Haas & Cummings, 1994, p. 139)

Many general hospitals opened psychiatric units because charges for such disorders were exempted from the Medicare DRG payment system. Not only were ADM services reimbursed on a fee-for-service basis, but psychiatric beds are less expensive to operate than are medical beds, and they can produce a higher margin of return on investment. Many of the vacant beds resulting from reduced medical admissions and lengths of stay for Medicare and private patients were profitably converted to psychiatric or substance abuse units. (Broskowski, 1994, p. 9)

This [review] has demonstrated (a) that cost problems in the delivery of mental health services are largely associated with the costs of inpatient, not of outpatient, care; (b) that the efficacy of inpatient treatment compared with outpatient alternatives is largely unproved and therefore closer to an experimental than a well-validated treatment; (c) that the costs of mental health care are largely attributable to a relatively small number of consumers of mental health services; and (d) that mental health benefits are largely designed in an inappropriate manner. (Lowman, 1994, p. 134)

Lowman (1994) noted that reviews of the outcome literature generally show that hospital-based treatment of psychological problems for adults, adolescents, and children rarely bests outpatient treatment. Lowman also observed that mental health benefits are typically more generous for inpatient options: at the time of his writing, only 50 percent of outpatient care was usually reimbursed, compared to 80 percent of inpatient care.

Kessler (1998) reported that while behavioral health claims accounted for only 3 to 4 percent of total medical claims during the 1960s and 1970s, in the 1970s the percentage began to increase. In the 1970s some privately owned psychiatric hospitals grew 20 to 25 percent annually with after-tax profits of 20 percent. New psychiatric hospitals were frequently opening and general hospitals increased their mental health services (cf. Silverman & Miller, 1994). By 1990 behavioral health care accounted for 10 percent of claims with some employers spending 20 to 25 percent on mental health. By 1998, however, behavioral health care had returned to its previous levels of accounting for only 3 to 4 percent of medical claims (Kessler, 1998). Nevertheless, some estimates of mental health problems in the general population indicate a much greater need for treatment. For example, some estimates place the number of American children with at least one significant mental health problem at 15 to 20 percent (e.g., Weisz, Huey, & Weersing, 1998).

Broskowski (1994) noted that over the past 50 years, hospital-based care has been the greatest contributor to increasing health costs. Hospitals billed insurance companies during this period on the basis of the cost of a procedure plus profit (often 15 percent). Insurers simply passed higher costs along to employers who provided tax-deductible health insurance to employers. Cummings and Sayama (1995) suggested that the government's introduction of Diagnosis Related Groups (DRGs) significantly changed this process. DRGs describe categories of illnesses that might be treated within a certain time frame. DRGs meant that Medicare and Medicaid reimbursement were based on the diagnosis of the patient instead of the previous cost plus profit. The result of DRGs, Cummings and Sayama maintained (1995, p. 19), was that:

> The federal government not only ushered in the era of managed care, but inadvertently launched the full-scale industrialization of health care. After 200 years as a cottage industry, health care began a rapid industrialization, with the blessing of those who pay the bills: the employers. Decades of laws forbidding the corporate practice of medicine or the proprietary ownership of hospitals, clinics, and health systems were either ignored or repealed.

Note that Cummings and Sayama (1995) use the word "ignored" to discuss corporate behavior in regard to existing laws and regulations. As we shall see later, some managed care companies ignore rules and regulations— even their own—when it benefits them.

History of behavioral managed care

The beginnings of managed care are typically marked with examples of early health care organizations (Fox, 1997), including:

- Western Clinic in Tacoma, Washington, which in 1910 offered medical services through its own providers for the rate of 50 cents per member per month.
- A farmers' cooperative health plan, started in 1929 in Elk City, Oklahoma, which charged farmers $50 per share to raise money for a new hospital where they could receive discounted medical care.
- The Kaiser Foundation Health Plans, begun in 1937 at the request of the Kaiser construction company to finance medical care for the workers and families building an aqueduct to transport water from the Colorado River to Los Angeles.

Fox (1997) noted that traditional health insurance is also of relatively recent origin. The beginnings of Blue Cross, for example, can be traced to a 1929 Baylor (Texas) Hospital agreement to provide prepaid care to 1,500 teachers. Fox (1997) also attributed the formation of other Blue Cross and Blue Shield plans during the Great Depression not to consumer demand, but to the desire of providers attempting to "protect and enhance patient revenues" (p. 4).

Davis (1998) noted that in the past 50 years numerous attempts have been made to change the cost, quality, and access to the U.S. health care system. The fee-for-service system was seen as providing the "wrong incentives" to physicians (Fox, 1997, p. 6). Although the recent proliferation of for-profit managed care organizations (MCOs) is the latest significant effort, the federal government has clearly had a significant hand in health policy, particularly as costs have risen for Medicare (Zarabozo & LeMasurier, 1997) and Medicaid (Hurley, Kirschner, & Bone, 1997).

In addition to introducing DRGs, the federal government has played a significant role in promoting the growth of HMOs. The federal HMO Act of 1973 provided $325 million over a five-year period to encourage the startup of new HMOs and the slowing of health care costs (Newman & Reed, 1996). The 1973 HMO act also allowed profit-oriented corporations to become involved in HMOs (DeLeon, VandenBos, & Bulatao, 1994) and set a precedent of defining mental health benefits as covering only crisis intervention and acute care (Kessler, 1998). Cummings and Sayama (1995) maintained that the federal HMO legislation was a response to the successful efforts of the American Medical Association to prevent capitated medicine (where payment is limited to a fixed amount per person in the plan). They indicated that the AMA had successfully lobbied state legislatures to oppose capitation and continue fee-for-service payments (where payment depends upon the service provided). The federal legislation "rendered all of this crippling state legislation irrelevant inasmuch as federally chartered HMOs were made exempt from most state statutes" (Cummings & Sayama, 1995, p. 18). Newman and Reed (1996) concluded that the law was so successful that "the pendulum seemed to have radically shifted away from an almost exclusive emphasis on treatment and services to a comparable singular focus on costs, financial issues, and economic resources in the provision of health care" (p. 14).

Pedulla and Rocke (1999) described the Employee Retirement Income Securities Act (ERISA) of 1974 as federal legislation designed to protect workers' retirement plans. However, ERISA also applied to plans that provided medical and other kinds of benefits to employees. And while ERISA applied to most plans, it did not cover employees of church, government institutions, or persons who purchased insurance as individuals. In health care, the primary effect of ERISA has been to prevent persons who have been denied treatment by their HMO from suing their insurer. Likewise, ERISA can prevent employees from suing for damages for injuries, obtaining external appeals of benefit denials, and seeking deadlines for urgent care decisions. Because the law was designed to "free employers subject to

ERISA from having to meet a patchwork quilt of differing state laws" (Pedulla & Rocke, 1999, p. 2), ERISA overrode all state laws regarding employee benefit plans. Pedulla and Rocke (1999) described ERISA as applying to fully insured plans (where the employer purchases an insurance policy that provides health care for employees) but not to self-insured plans (where the employer directly pays health care costs and hence is not in the insurance business per se). Pedulla and Rocke (1999) concluded:

> In short, ERISA has often blocked patients injured by managed care and other health care plans from holding these plans legally accountable for their treatment decision making. At times the law precludes patients and providers outright from obtaining any state-based relief to which other plaintiffs in similar situations would be entitled. Further . . . ERISA has repeatedly been used as a procedural device to delay legal action. (p. 18)

Three phases of behavioral managed care

Another way to examine the history of managed care is to describe the economic and market forces affecting the behavioral health care companies. Kessler (1998), a CEO of one of the first companies in the managed behavioral health care field, provided such a perspective. He believes that three distinct phases have occurred during the transition to managed care dominance in mental health insurance. Each of these is described here.

Phase 1

During the first phase in the mid-1980s, Kessler (1998) indicated that the domination of the health care market by traditional health insurers such as Blue Cross began to shift to HMOs. He noted that "since HMOs generally placed price above other considerations, the major goal in this phase of managed behavioral health care was to maximize savings" (p. 155). Notably, the primary strategy employed to reach this goal was to cut access to services. Kessler noted that some HMOs made facilities difficult to reach; in one HMO, only one substance abuse program was available, about four hours away by car in another state. HMOs also offered only a small panel (i.e., approved group) of providers, hiring providers who shared the HMO's philosophy and accepted the accompanying limits. Naturally, the majority of providers rebelled against these efforts.

Phase 2

Kessler (1998) described the second phase, in the years around 1990, as focused on large employers, now identified as the target market of the behavioral managed care companies. Despite initial resistance, managed care companies began to convince large firms to separate or carve out behavioral health from other medical services. They did this by persuading companies—with the help of professional associations and patient advocacy groups (Newman & Reed, 1996)—that behavioral health was distinct and required specialized expertise. Kessler (1998) maintains that this process was further assisted by (a) publicity about psychiatric hospital scandals in which mental health patients were exploited and (b) CEOs of major companies who decided to become actively involved with the problem of increasing health care costs (cf. Gottlieb, 1995).

The result, Kessler believes, was that large firms wanted some degree of cost control and a minimization of complaints from patients. Kessler suggests that while this influenced managed care companies to use more open panels of providers, they now devised another method of controlling costs: demanding deep discounts from providers. Professionals began to provide discounts of 20 to 25 percent while hospitals reduced their charges by 25 to 35 percent. Kessler maintains that these changes meant higher client satisfaction since the pain had been transferred from beneficiaries to providers.

Phase 3

Kessler (1998) suggested that a third phase (mid-1990s to current) has been marked by the consolidation of managed care companies. The large traditional insurers are gone from this market or about to be extinct; large national managed care companies own almost all significant behavioral health care companies. The target market in this third phase moved to small firms and the public sector, with the possibility of "doubling the industry's revenues in 5 years" (Kessler, 1998, p. 157).

By this time Kessler declared that "Provider resistance was broken, and managed behavioral health companies found a seemingly inexhaustible supply of providers to replace those who wouldn't accept new, lower reimbursement rates" (p. 157). The supply of mental health professionals was greater than the reduced need for providers used by managed care. Kessler (1998) reported that the number of licensed outpatient providers had grown geometrically over the past three decades as social workers and psychologists won legal battles to bill insurers directly. The number of licensed therapists (e.g., social workers, psychologists, and psychiatrists) jumped from 80,000 to more than 300,000. This pool enabled managed care companies to find a sufficient number of providers willing to implement their policies. One of the results, Kessler (1998) reported, is that the incomes of providers in these professions are in a steep decline. Managed care companies also need fewer mental health professionals since these companies tend to decrease the ratio of mental health staff to insured members (cf. Scheffler & Ivey, 1998).

Discounts grew to 40 to 45 percent for professionals and 50 to 65 percent for hospitals. In some cities all professionals are currently being paid $40 to $45 for a 45-minute session (Kessler, 1998). Sauber (1997b) reported the fee is now under $25 in major markets such as Los Angeles and San Francisco.

Three phases?

VanLeit (1996) argued that for most managed care companies, there have been only two phases. In the first phase—where we believe many managed care companies remain—extensive utilization review is used to control costs. Utilization review refers to the examination of clinical information, by representatives of the health plan, to determine the medical necessity of services (i.e., services necessary and appropriate for the diagnosis and treatment of medical conditions) and insure their cost-effectiveness. Utilization reviewers in this phase often use criteria that are kept secret from clinicians, leading to "tremendous distrust, paranoia, and hostility between managed care companies and providers" (VanLeit, 1996, p. 430). One health plan, for example, authorizes 10 sessions for clients but does not inform therapists that those sessions must be used by a certain date.

In phase 2 companies still try to hold down costs but pay more attention to quality and effectiveness of care. These companies focus on outcome measurement, share utilization criteria and standards of care, and shift the financial risk (through capitation) to providers. While most companies provide consumers and therapists with extensive literature on their commitment to quality, we see little solid evidence that managed care companies or administrators in other settings who use managed care methods have shifted to this phase. Instead, cost dominates all other factors, with a host of resulting problems.

The consequences of managed care

While HMOs have stopped rapid increases in costs, they have also created additional problems and done little to address other important health care issues. The following brief list includes topics that we will further discuss in subsequent chapters.

Lack of adequate health care

The most serious problem concerns the 40 million plus Americans who lack adequate health care. For example, a 1995 national telephone survey of 3,993 randomly selected persons by the National Opinion

Research Center found that nearly one-third reported (a) being unin-sured, (b) did not get medical care at a time they needed it, or (c) had problems paying medical bills (Birenbaum & Cohen, 1998). Some had thought that cost savings would translate into wider insurance coverage because the insurance would be more affordable (cf. Daniels, Light, & Caplan, 1996, p. 4). However, the money made or saved by managed care companies has generally not been used to insure more people.

As managed care companies limit the number of providers to save costs, the sickest may get the worst treatment at the hands of the remaining providers who will see them. Sauber (1997b, p. 16) concluded that "the bot-tom line is that managed care often buys little in the way of savings but may cost dearly in terms of quality of care—occasionally with tragic results." Similarly, Broskowski (1994) noted that although some research has documented a decrease in inappropriate care and fraudulent practices among providers, "improvements in the quality of care (an often-neglected managed care variable) have been harder to demonstrate" (p. 12).

An obsession with cost

As we have noted, the most significant and obvious change is how the focus has switched away from providing the best services to cost (Newman & Reed, 1996). The cost emphasis manifests itself in a variety of ways across settings. In counseling, for example, the cost emphasis typically translates into brief therapy as well as denial of and delays of services to clients and payments to providers.

A recent report examining the health plans of 1,017 U.S. employers (Rabasca, 1999) found that over the past 10 years health plans cut mental health benefits proportionally more than other types of health care:

- The value of the average mental health benefit has been cut from $154.08 per covered individual in 1988 to $69.61 in 1997.

- Spending on behavioral health equaled 3.1 percent of all health care benefit dollars in 1997, compared to 6.2 percent in 1988.

- Annual limits on outpatient visits rose to 57 percent of plans in 1998 from 48 percent in 1997. The most common limit is 20 visits per year, imposed by about one-third of the plans with limits. As we will see later, these numbers actually underestimate the limits imposed by health plans.

- More plans charge a separate co-payment for mental health care. These co-pays may be significantly higher than those charged for other services.

- More plans limit inpatient psychiatric care.

Agency hardships

The *zeitgeist* of slashing funding for mental health can also be found in the public sector. Over the past decade many agencies that receive funding from state, county, or city governments have seen disproportionate cuts. Agencies face the challenge of trying to provide basic services while faced with the task of raising money from other sources. The typical result is an increased workload for all staff, fewer administrators and support staff, and pressure to dismiss counselors seen as unproductive. Agency counselors who see too many long-term clients or too few clients who pay directly or through insurance reimbursement are likely to be considered unproductive. Agencies may also lack the money or expertise to obtain or upgrade computer equipment and software to perform tasks such as client record-keeping and billing. And when managed care companies delay claims payments for months, agencies must find ways to meet their payrolls.

Types of services and who delivers them

One study examined the effects of managed care over a four-year period in the 1990s on community mental health agencies in the state of New York. Cypres, Landsberg, and Spellmann (1997) surveyed directors of 562 agencies who provided outpatient services. Cypres et al. (1997) found that agencies reported providing less open-ended psychotherapy and psychological testing and more brief therapy, medication, crisis intervention, and substance abuse treatment. Decreases in doctoral-level psychologists and increases in psychiatrists, nurses, and masters- or bachelor-level counselors accompanied these alterations in intervention modes.

De-emphasis on psychiatric hospitalization

Kessler (1998) provided data to illustrate the extent of some of the changes in hospitals. First, the number of psychiatric inpatient hospital days per 1,000 lives declined from 150 in 1983 (traditional insurers) to 75 in 1990 (employer carve-outs) to 25 in 1998 (HMOs). Kessler (1998) expects the number to continue to decrease and says the changes have "devastated the psychiatric hospital industry" (p. 158). While a strong case can be made to transition more care from inpatient to outpatient settings, a need for a strong inpatient network in every locale is likely to remain for such problems as substance abuse and chronic mental illness.

Increase in paperwork and administrative costs

Another problem exacerbated by managed care is increased paperwork for clients and clinicians. Reuters reported that over the past 25 years the percentage of health care workers doing mostly paperwork rose from

18.1 percent to 27.1 percent in 1993. While the proportion of doctors and nurses who care for patients fell over that period, the number of health care administrators grew by 692 percent. Sauber (1997b) concluded that managed care adds "bureaucracy to an already bloated system" (p. 16), while others estimate that 24 percent of the amount spent on health care goes toward administration (Center for Health Economics Research, 1993).

The almost universal experience of clinicians is that managed care wastes a tremendous amount of their time. In the managed care system clinicians are routinely expected to spend hours on such tasks as waiting on the phone to reach company representatives, preparing justifications for treatment, conducting utilization reviews, and rescheduling utilization review meetings cancelled by the company. External or utilization reviews are a particular onerous portion of the paperwork problem for counselors; here the therapist must justify her or his rationale for providing services to a particular client. Mechanic (1997, p. 104) noted that "at its best . . . external case management can be collaborative and constructive, but it also presents opportunities for intrusive interference, disagreements, and conflict." Providers have been estimated to spend between 15 and 22 percent of their budget to handle the administrative procedures required by managed care (Daniels et al., 1996).

The paperwork becomes even more tedious at the agency level. For example, an agency that wishes to enter into a contract with a managed care company typically must submit an application for the agency as a whole as well as complete the credentialing process for each therapist employed at the agency. One agency administrator described the process to us as a "nightmare."

Another characteristic of many managed care companies is that they are constantly changing their procedures and provider requirements. As one therapist told us, "Managed care companies change their procedures more often than most people change underwear." Again, the problem is compounded at the agency level, where procedural changes can affect hundreds of clients.

Given this context, it is not surprising that administrative costs are higher in a managed care system for both insurers and providers. Daniels et al. (1996) reported that in New Jersey managed care companies have administrative costs between 14 and 20 percent, compared to 4.5 percent for traditional health plans in that state. Managed care costs often include marketing, consultants, and substantial salaries for managers.

Training opportunities

Training opportunities for students in the helping professions have been described as being under siege (Spiggle & Hughes, 1998; but see Constantine

& Gloria, 1998, for a different view). The most dramatic effects of managed care have been to decrease or eliminate training programs in some agencies (Brooks & Riley, 1998; Davis, 1998).

Graduate students who attempt to generate financial support at their practica agencies are likely to find that managed care companies will not pay them—ostensibly because they are not licensed (American Psychological Association, 1998). Similarly, supervision time cannot be reimbursed under managed care. Our experience is that a lack of a professional degree has become another tactic in managed care's strategy to deny services. In addition, most managed care companies have little or no stake in training mental health providers.

Changes in training opportunities because of managed care can also be subtler. In our doctoral program, students report that at some practica sites they have difficulty obtaining enough clients or clients of a certain type. One student, for example, was able to see only clients who carried traditional Medicaid at an agency because managed care would not reimburse her for their clients. Traditional Medicaid clients (as opposed to Medicaid covered by managed care) were relatively few, however, and the student had to travel to an additional practicum site to obtain a sufficient number of clients. Another student desired experience with elderly clients, but the practicum agency saw only elderly enrolled in a special seniors program at a managed care company—which wouldn't reimburse students. As this student said, "I could have seen elderly self-pay clients, but there aren't any!"

Donner (1998) listed other training problems associated with field sites affected by managed care, including:

- Decreased ability to provide training in long-term mental health services. Short-term therapy is now the dominant modality.
- Stressed staff members seeing students as burdens, rather than assets. Staff who provide excellent supervision may do so at their own expense.

Ethical and legal difficulties

Managed care can lead to increased liability for clinicians because clinicians may have an ethical and legal obligation to appeal treatment denials (Sauber, 1997b). For example, the court case of *Wickline v. State of California* (1987) made it the provider's responsibility to push insurance companies for adequate care (Newman & Bricklin, 1994). Clinicians also have a responsibility to insure that clients have continued professional support once the managed care companies terminate sessions.

At the other extreme, capitation may create ethical concerns for some providers. Some managed care companies may offer providers a flat fee for treatment, regardless of the number of sessions. In such situations the counselor now has dual roles (a) provide the best possible care to the client, versus (b) provide the least expensive (i.e., time-consuming) care for the managed care company. As one reviewer of this book noted, "Some demands of MCOs may be legal but unethical." A similar situation faces utilization reviewers who see themselves as patient advocates (Anderson, Berlant, Mauch, & Maloney, 1997) but must prioritize the MCO's demands for cost control.

Confidentiality issues also arise: The information required by managed care companies may violate the privacy of clients, and clinicians cannot guarantee the confidentiality of this information once it leaves their office. We provide more specific examples in the following chapters.

The psychotherapy factory

While counselors historically have felt ambivalent about the application of the medical model to their work, they now must deal with the business model. Managed care companies consider counseling and psychotherapy part of a health care "industry" complete with the vocabulary and methods thereof. Sauber (1997b, p. xii–xiv) summarized the trends:

> We are now faced with control of mental health by business managers and investors, the exploitation of inexpensive labor in the form of reduced provider fees, and the use of lesser-credentialed counselors and mental health technicians, standardized cookbooks of care where covered lives are channeled through predetermined treatment; mass delivery vehicles, such as group therapy; computerized assessment and treatment checklists; routine dispension of psychotropic medications by nonpsychiatric physicians; mergers and acquisitions leading to semi-monopolies; and a mass exodus by private practitioners out of the profession.

Summary

Business and government have collaborated in their attempts to stop steady increases in health care costs. By bolstering the development of managed care through federal legislation and the push of most employees into HMOs, managed care companies now wield extraordinary influence in the delivery of health care. In the mental health area, managed care companies have focused almost exclusively on cost, cutting access to services and drastically reducing fees to providers. Such reductions have been applied to both outpatient and inpatient services, despite the fact that most mental health costs are associated with inpatient care.

The Parameters of Managed Mental Health Care

This chapter addresses the specific ways that managed mental health care has impacted on the practice of outpatient psychotherapy (also see Richardson & Austad, 1994). Prior to introduction of managed care, counseling sessions, documentation, and the counseling process largely remained private between the counselor and the client. All of these components were designed to meet the needs of the counselor, agency, and client. If third-party reimbursement (i.e., traditional indemnity health insurance) was available, it was considered the responsibility of the client to see that the company paid the counselor's fee. The specifics of treatment were considered "none of the insurance company's business."

Many counselors had been trained to value autonomy and regarded any outside influence on the therapy process as an intrusion. Ethical practice required that all counseling be the best possible (e.g., American Psychological Association, 1992; American Rehabilitation Counseling Association, 1987; American School Counselor Association, 1992; Association for Specialists in Group Work, 1989; Canadian Psychological Association, 1991; Herlihy & Corey, 1996; National Association of School Psychologists, 1992; National Association of Social Workers, 1994; National Board for Certified Counselors, 1989; National Career Development Association, 1987). Thus, the outside evaluation of the practices surrounding counseling seemed superfluous. Although researchers were busily evaluating the overall efficacy of counseling (e.g., Lambert & Hill, 1994), specific violations of ethical or competent practice were usually detected only if a client reported the counselor. The bodies responsible for licensing a counselor had the power to discipline, but (outside of instances of fraud) third-party payers typically did not.

Today, most offices and agencies have complex, often contradictory, and frequently expensive requirements regarding how the office must run. Managed care companies feel not only entitled, but obligated to dictate just how their "providers" should conduct themselves both in session and in the office. This chapter will attempt to describe how a typical counselor must navigate this confusing web of requirements.

Assume most provider panels are restricted

The majority of managed care provider panels restrict membership on the panel beyond the requirement that the provider possesses adequate credentials (Kessler, 1998). Counselors should investigate which restrictions apply to which companies in which areas. Just because a company limits membership in one area does not necessarily mean it will limit membership in the same way somewhere else. However, we describe common types of limitations.

Geographic limitations

Perhaps the most common limitation is the location of your office. Many companies limit the number of mental health clinicians in the most popular areas to practice. Conversely, the least popular areas (e.g., rural and some urban settings) may be wide open. In fact, a counselor may have more leeway to practice as he or she wishes in some of the areas under-represented by panel members in mental health.

Sometimes location can be used to the clinician's advantage to gain membership on a panel:

> One therapist was quite puzzled to learn that she had been admitted to a panel to which the majority of her colleagues had been denied. In fact, she had been allowed to join the panel when many colleagues who had previously counseled clients for this company for years had been thrown off. While she would have preferred to believe that her edge lay in her brilliant skills, she knew better. Her advantage was the fact that she had recently joined (on a three-hour per week basis) a rural practice. That, coupled with a full-time urban practice, did the trick.

On the other hand, the limits of geography can absurdly limit a clinician's mobility. In some cases, a move down the street to another office has resulted in the clinician's removal from a panel. Particularly if the managed care company is looking for a reason to downsize or drop a troublesome panel member, the address change can provide a convenient reason. Thus, do not assume that your clients will simply be able to see you at your new office location. If you have the option of choosing to move or not, you will be well advised to check with each company prior to your move.

Starting out

Because many panels are closed to new providers soon after the managed care company moves into a new region, clinicians with recently obtained licenses and/or degrees may have difficulty starting to build a practice. Likewise, it is often difficult even for experienced clinicians to build a practice in a new city or region. Several options do exist, however. Often a clinician with a relatively rare and/or high demand specialization (i.e., neuropsychology or treatment of disorders of infancy) may make some progress with panels that are generally closed. As mentioned, practicing in an underrepresented area may also help.

Joining a group

Many newcomers join group practices or agencies that have group panel membership (Grossberg, 1997). The clinician is then admitted to the panel because he or she is working for a group with a negotiated contract with the managed care company. Be advised, however, if one leaves the group or agency, the panel membership is rarely transportable.

Groups offer many advantages, particularly if one is starting out or new to a region. Groups often have established reputations in a community and with the managed care companies. This allows for a steady referral system that is more difficult for the individual. Expenses such as marketing, billing services, secretarial staff, and office space can be shared. A staff with diverse areas of experience and expertise allows for efficient consultation and smooth referral when necessary. Some managed care companies will only panel members of group practices or agencies. In fact, some mental health experts predict the demise of the solo practitioner (Moldawsky, 1990). On the other hand, group practices may limit the ability to practice with autonomy. Often a counselor is required to conform to the group practice's procedures for therapy as well as for office policy:

> A group practice has a 24-hour cancellation policy. Clients are charged the full session fee for sessions not cancelled prior to the 24 hours. While this policy is common in private practice, most clinicians use some discretion in its implementation. A young clinician in this group practice was forced (against his therapeutic judgement) to charge his client for the missed session when the client accompanied her mother to the emergency room of the local hospital rather than attend the session.

Some new counselors hope to join group practices to gain admission to the closed provider panels with the plan to work for the group and later open a practice of their own. Do not assume that it will be possible to take the panel memberships along to the new practice. Counselors with 10 years experience with a given group practice and managed care company have been summarily dismissed from the panel after they have left the group.

The financial incentives and disincentives for joining a group practice to gain membership to panels is also complicated. It is often true that a counselor working for him or herself will pay less in overhead and office expenses than the same counselor might if he or she paid a percentage of practice income (often as high as 50 to 70 percent, paid to the group's executive staff and for administrative expenses). Some groups, however, are able to negotiate increased fees or other special favors (e.g., easier utilization review) with the managed care companies.

Some clinicians have attempted to take the advantages from both individual and group dealings with managed care by forming their own IPAs. Individuals in these type of groups retain more of their treatment and financial autonomy, but negotiate with and market to managed care companies as a more powerful group.

Regardless of the type of group, some managed care companies now emphatically state that they will not accept counselors in individual practice for panel membership. Deciding to pursue an individual practice and work with managed care may not be an option in the future.

Effects on clients

Although this section has focused primarily on the effects of panel restrictions on therapists, clients can clearly experience major hassles in their attempts to obtain mental health care. Expect that many of your new clients will be frustrated by the time they finally reach you:

A psychologist reported receiving a number of referrals for neuropsychological testing from medical doctors in one health plan. However, the psychologist is not on the plan's panel. Each patient calls the plan and is told to ask their physician to make an out-of-plan referral. However, these referrals are subsequently rejected by the plan, whose representatives then tell patients to use a psychologist on their panel. One patient paid out-of-pocket for testing rather than wait an additional two months to be seen by a panel provider.

A patient with an eating disorder called her insurer to request a therapist with this specialty. The managed care company, however, reported that they simply provide provider names and do not know provider specialty areas.

Applying for panel membership
with a managed care company

The application process varies widely from managed care company to managed care company. A few companies have a relatively straightforward process designed to establish that the clinician's credentials, experience, and availability are sufficient to provide therapy services. Many application requirements, however, are cumbersome, detailed, and time-consuming.

The National Committee for Quality Assurance (NCQA) is an organization developed by the managed care industry to set minimal standards for managed care companies. Because most companies desire NCQA accreditation, provider applications will require information to meet these basic standards. Most often, the information required as part of the application process is far more detailed.

Typically, the counselor will be required to show proof of licensure, degree, and current malpractice coverage. Regarding malpractice, check to see how much coverage is required; many companies specify the amount. Many companies will not accept a provider that is not licensed. Some companies require proof that the counselor's office is covered by accident insurance. Most require information regarding the therapist's malpractice history, drug and alcohol abuse, mental illness, and significant legal history. Other common requirements include proof of internship (for psychologists), Drug Enforcement Administration certificate and Controlled Substance Registration certificate (for physicians), and hospital affiliations and board certification (for psychiatrists). The authors have also been required to submit letters of recommendation from other professionals, syllabi from courses taken in graduate training, and copies of facesheets from all years of insurance malpractice coverage for the past 10 years. Often photocopies of documents such as licenses are not accepted. Originals must be ordered and sent.

Companies sometimes have their own ideas regarding what constitutes areas of specialization in an area of counseling. A counselor who reports that she or he specializes in sexual abuse survivors, for example, may be required to submit documentation specified by the company (e.g., three course syllabi and two years supervised experience) to qualify to treat that population. Documentation of continuing education may be required. If the therapist practices in a state without required continuing education, it is useful to request official proof of attendance at continuing education conferences for submission with managed care applications.

Finally, information regarding office hours, secretarial staff, crisis availability (e.g., Do you carry a beeper? Have an answering service?), accessibility for clients with disabilities, and languages other than English may be required. The company may ask for the name(s) and phone numbers of psychiatrists with whom you work. Often you will be required to outline a plan for coverage of clients when you are out of the area or indisposed for a length of time. Because the company will pay only panel members, coverage arrangements must be made with other panel members. Some companies require familiarity and comfort with brief treatment models and a personal statement outlining therapeutic approach.

Understanding managed care provider contracts

David Nevin, Ph.D., past president of the New York State Psychological Association, once described the climate surrounding clinicians contracting with managed care companies as akin to the pre-labor union days of the 1920s and 30s when yellow-dog contracts were prevalent. Essentially, these were contracts designed for and by employers with the main or sole purpose of meeting the employers' needs. Because the labor force was so plentiful and people so desperate to work, an individual who did not like the terms of the contract was simply advised to "take it or leave it." Plenty of additional workers were eager to sign the contract, no matter how unfair.

Managed care companies have significantly limited provider panels and restricted third-party benefits. At the same time, several of the mental health professions have significantly increased the number of degreed individuals they are graduating (Schamess & Lightburn, 1998). The increase in therapists and decrease in resources for therapy—client need for therapy does not figure into this equation—has resulted in a "yellow dog" situation. Few providers have the ability to change the contracts written by the managed care companies.

It is important to read thoroughly all contracts before signing them. While that sounds obvious, it becomes difficult to do this completely when receiving another contract from some new or renamed company every few weeks. Also, most contracts are many pages long and written in legalese. Do not let this deter you from reading the contracts thoroughly; you do not want to find yourself legally responsible for terms that are unacceptable. If you have access to an attorney, consider sharing questionable contracts with her or him for advice before signing.

Some of the more common problematic clauses found in managed mental health contracts include the following (cf. Giles, 1993).

Hold harmless

Most HMOs require the clinician to sign a statement releasing the company from liability should the clinician be held responsible for damages as a function of the services provided by the clinician. The therapist must carry his/her own malpractice coverage. On the surface this appears to make sense. The counselor should be responsible for substandard practice. However, it is important to examine the clause carefully to ensure that the HMO is not indemnified against its own limits on practice. For example, in *Wickline v. State of California* (1987), the provider was held liable for the HMO's decision to limit hospitalization even when the provider recommended further treatment. The court ruled that the provider did not appeal the denial aggressively enough. There have since been a number of legal cases addressing the issue of provider responsibility and HMO cost-containment strategies. The area remains murky both legally and ethically.

Limited reimbursement

This typically refers to the company's responsibility to pay the provider. If for any reason the company does not pay the provider for legitimate services, the client is not responsible for payment and the provider must continue to provide services covered in the contract. While the provider still may pursue legal action to recover payment from the company, the cost of retaining legal counsel and going to court against a large and powerful company is often not worth the money recovered.

> A not-for-profit community mental health agency is owed thousands of dollars in back payments from a nationally known managed care company. All claims submitted since the new company took over management of a particular insurance benefit have remained unpaid. Although the state requires that a legitimate and properly documented claim be paid within 45 days of submission, the claims are currently 135 days overdue. The agency has been unable to pay some of its staff and expenses. While legal action is possible, the agency cannot wait for the legal process and has an ethical responsibility to continue to care for the clients in question.

Gag clauses

These clauses have become less common over time. Essentially they prevent the therapist from discussing with the client treatment possibilities not covered by the insurance plan. The therapist is not free to discuss or recommend treatments that the therapist feels may benefit the client if the client's insurance company does not cover it. This leaves the client with the impression that the best treatment is the one covered by the company. In mental health this most often means an emphasis on short-term behavioral or medication-based treatment.

Treatment protocols

Some contracts specify limits of mental health treatment protocols covered. Some treatment approaches are covered and some are not:

> A psychologist was denied permission to address parenting skills with a depressed single mother coping with her ADHD child. Parenting skills were not a covered treatment in the mother's insurance plan.
>
> A therapist was denied permission for marital therapy for a couple. While the wife was eligible for treatment for her depression, the treatment plan could not include couples therapy because it was not a covered treatment benefit. The wife and therapist both attributed her depression to the difficult marital situation. The managed care company's representative suggested that the woman obtain "good insurance" if she wanted to receive the marital therapy recommended for her care.

Behaviors outside of the contract

Some contracts specify behaviors required of the therapist even after the client's benefits are exhausted or not in force. For example, the company may prohibit the therapist from continuing to treat a client on his or her own once the company has denied further treatment. Continuing treatment at a reduced fee or at the client's expense might be prohibited even if both client and therapist agree it is necessary. Other contracts require that the therapist turn over to the company all case notes, even those for counseling conducted prior to insurance coverage by the current company.

Termination without cause

A common clause states that the company may remove a therapist from its provider panel without revealing the reason. This clause frightens many therapists away from pushing for the full services needed by clients. They are fearful that they will be labeled problematic by the company and removed from the panel.

Appointment response time

Some contracts require the therapist to guarantee a quick first appointment for any member. The time frame usually ranges from two days to one week for a client not in crisis. Crisis clients often must be seen the same day. This requirement has the potential to be quite beneficial for the client in eliminating unnecessarily long waits for needed treatment. However, it creates a serious double-bind for therapists and (eventually) for clients. Because the panels are kept small, a therapist on a given panel may have many clients from that insurance plan. If the therapist is on several panels, he or she may be so busy that it is difficult to take on more clients without compromising the care of the clients currently being treated. Meanwhile, qualified therapists not admitted to the panels may have plenty of free time to see someone new immediately.

Pay attention to your income expectations

This guideline holds particularly for professionals in private practice, but may also apply in settings such as agencies and hospitals. The reimbursement fees for providing services to managed care clients vary from company to company, area to area, and over time. Many companies have reduced the fees paid to all providers from the fees agreed to when contracts were first signed. Counselors need to think about the lowest fees or salary they are willing to accept before leaving a managed care company; fees may continue to decrease.

> A therapist received notice that a major managed care company in the state had lowered its fees for licensed psychologists by 21 percent. The counselor's practice included a fair number of clients carrying this insurance, so income for these clients dropped an immediate 21 percent with no other changes in how therapy was managed. The company did not notify the clients of this change.

In the past, fees differed according to level of training (e.g., M.A. vs. Ph.D.), but the gap is steadily narrowing. Many companies no longer differentiate fee schedules based on level of training for providing the same service. This impacts both independent clinicians and salaried staff at agencies and hospitals. Many can no longer afford to pay higher salaries to doctoral clinicians. In fact, some agencies hire only beginning masters-level counselors because they cannot afford experienced counselors or professionals with doctoral degrees.

At the same time that fees are decreasing, overhead costs are rising (Yenney, 1994). Some companies require a receptionist/secretary to ensure quick and easy access to the mental health professional. Other requirements may include an answering service, electronic billing capability, and beeper accessibility.

Even if a secretary is not a managed care company requirement, most clinicians find this a necessity. Billing and utilization review procedures have become so detailed and cumbersome that the therapist rarely has time to devote to such matters. It is common to remain on the phone line of a company's billing office for 10 to 15 minutes before the call is answered. Often, voice mail is reached and a message must be left. A full-time secretary is needed to receive the return call or make repeated calls since the company may not make an effort to respond.

Managed care companies may need repeated prompting to pay legitimate claims. Errors in the direction of denying claims seem all too common. The bill is filed, a month or two passes before payment is rejected, the company is called to correct the error, and another month or two passes before the error is corrected and the bill paid.

> One clinician reports that it is rare when she does not have two or three outstanding bills from managed care companies that are over six months old. Many require repeated phone calls to the company. Despite promises from the company's billing clerk to correct the error, the claim is rejected again and again. The therapist's secretary can spend many hours trying to recover just one claim. The financially smaller claims are not worth the cost of the secretarial time and are just written off.

> A therapist noted a history of denied and delayed claims with a particular health plan. They denied claims if they are billed 90 days after services are provided but take as long as 210 days to pay.

> Many health plans do not hire sufficient numbers of utilization reviewers or employees in claims departments to handle the workload. A therapist's calls to an insurer who had not paid in several months were finally answered by a clerk who indicated that she had been on maternity leave and returned to find 175 unpaid claims waiting for her attention.

> A therapist saw a client for 10 sessions over a five-month period. The health plan paid for 10 sessions, but then took back payment for 9 of the 10 sessions because the ID number on the referral form from the physician was wrong by one number (the physician's office had been using this incorrect number for years). A corrected number and bill was sent to the insurer but no repayment was made until numerous phone calls were made and four months had passed.

Managed care companies make considerable money on the interest of funds acquired by delaying payment claims. The American Psychological Association (1999) conducted an analysis of potential interest income that managed care companies could make while claims are delayed. If denied claims had to proceed through an appeals process, as proposed in one version of health care legislation, insurance companies could generate interest income of up to $280 million each year if as few as 1 percent of claims were first denied and then reversed on appeal.

Co-payments

The client's portion of the financial responsibility for psychotherapy when a managed care company is covering the service is called the co-payment (Giles, 1993). While clients are usually familiar with the requirement to provide a co-payment when they use their coverage, they are often unprepared for the size of the mental health co-payment. This co-pay may differ significantly from the fee paid for an office visit to a physician and can be as high as 50 percent of the reimbursement fee to the therapist. This fee may make therapy difficult to afford, even for those with several approved sessions from their company. Because the therapist cannot charge the insurance companies different fees for the same service to different clients, she or he cannot reduce the co-payment to a client in need (e.g., Sands, Cullen, & Higuchi, 1996).

Some plans start with a relatively low co-payment and then increase it after a designated number of sessions (e.g., five). A frequently given rationale for this discrepancy is that therapeutic change happens best if there is personal sacrifice from the client in order to participate in therapy. Clients unwilling to pay more for therapy must not find it important enough to warrant the financial sacrifice. Instead, Blackwell, Gutmann, and Gutmann (1988) found that utilization rates for clients covered by a prepaid mental health plan were no higher than for clients paying for therapy themselves.

Clinics and agencies

Clients often seek treatment at a mental health clinic or agency with the hope that the services can be adjusted according to financial need. However, agencies and clinics that accept private insurance cannot reduce the company's co-payment any more than a private practitioner can (cf. Sands, Cullen, & Higuchi, 1996). Once the accepted insurance has been exhausted, however, the clinic or agency may be able to set a fee that the client can afford so that therapy can continue.

As funding for mental health services to clinics and agencies has shifted from public sources to private insurance, clinicians in agencies have been placed in an even more difficult position. Traditionally, these settings have been equipped to care for the chronically and/or high-need mentally ill client. Yet, if they use reimbursement from managed care companies, they are subject to the same limits and restrictions as the private practitioner. Services traditionally provided at clinics that are not part of the managed care contract must be eliminated or another funding source obtained.

As clinics and agencies scramble to meet the often contradictory requirements of public funding sources, managed care companies, communities, and clients, therapists are asked to cope with more difficult situations for less pay. Private clinicians may be more likely to refer chronic or difficult clients to agencies rather than work with them under managed care. Sadly, some private therapists work with difficult clients until the managed care benefit is exhausted or the company refuses further care, and then refer them to a clinic. The client suffers discontinuity of care and the clinic is left to pick up the ball. Recognizing this, some clinics may refuse services to clients who have already used some or all of their private insurance.

Be aware of the limits on the amount of therapy

Almost all managed care companies place limits on the amount of treatment (Giles, 1993; Haas & Cummings, 1994). The limits vary both in rigor and visibility. Some of the more common ways of limiting amount of treatment are described. For each client you see, be familiar with the limits so that you and your client do not receive an abrupt and counter-therapeutic disruption of your work together.

Medical necessity

This limit is virtually ubiquitous in the managed care era. It usually requires that the client meet diagnostic criteria for a DSM-IV or ICD-9 disorder (American Psychiatric Association, 1994). A client that wishes to use therapy to "self-actualize," "understand myself better," or "grow as a person," will likely be denied coverage if she or he does not have symptoms that fit a DSM-IV diagnosis. The medical model of mental illness and psychotherapeutic interventions is the only model considered.

Even when the DSM is consulted, some of the categories may be excluded as not being a "covered benefit." A common set of exclusions include the V Codes (DSM-IV), which are defined as conditions that are a focus of attention or treatment but are not attributable to any mental disorders. For example, a client may have enough symptoms to qualify for a diagnosis of Dysthymic Disorder and also have significant marital problems that directly affect his symptoms. Under many managed care contracts the therapist can help the client with dysthymic symptoms (including working out the marital problems with the spouse present), but cannot directly say she or he is treating the marital problems. Marital problems are covered in the DSM-IV as a V Code and often not covered directly by managed care. Of course, if the client does not have enough symptoms to meet a DSM-IV disorder but is still troubled by marital conflict, the therapy will not be covered.

Even when treatment is medically necessary, managed care companies may not respond quickly to requests for treatment they tend not to support:

> A psychologist requested authorization to administer an MMPI to evaluate suicidal ideation and masked depression in a client. He called twice and followed up with a letter. Despite the issue of potential suicide, the health plan did not respond to the request until 2 1/2 months had passed. The plan approved the request for testing.

Managed care companies may also throw obstacles in the way of beginning clearly needed treatments:

> Although arrangements had already been made through the primary care physician (PCP) for medication, the health plan mandated an alcohol assessment and psychiatric consultation for an 18-year-old patient. When his parents called the health plan to make these arrangements, the plan said the patient himself had to make the call because he was an adult. The therapist noted that the patient was depressed, substance-abusing, and failing school; expecting him to make these arrangements was unrealistic. The therapist called the company and after much arguing, the plan relented and provided authorization without the patient calling.

Medically appropriate

An important criterion for determining coverage for psychotherapy is the company's definition of medically appropriate treatment. This definition can include the very reasonable limit that the treatment must fit the client problem. Thus, a company may be reluctant to pay for Rogerian therapy for a cocaine-addicted client who comes to sessions high.

The managed care companies have, however, increasingly limited the types of therapeutic interventions they consider medically appropriate. Allen (1996) makes an important observation regarding treatment of psychological problems:

> Whatever is not tangible or visible is less understandable to people. A broken leg or a bullet wound, something that we can see or touch, is more comprehensible than something like anxiety or depression which is not visible or touchable. For most people—including government and insurance policy makers—psychiatric signs and symptoms are less comprehensible, less real. (p. 17)

Some counselors believe that this bias underlies the current trend of exempting "medical treatments" from utilization review, but retaining current utilization review procedures for psychotherapeutic interventions.

Because the focus tends to be on addressing signs and symptoms, behavioral and cognitive-behavioral interventions may be favored or required. It is important for any therapist working in a managed care environment today to be familiar with the language and methods of these interventions.

Crisis intervention

One method for limiting the amount of outpatient psychotherapy covered by a managed care company is to cover crisis or acute therapy only (Richardson & Austad, 1994). The definition of this kind of therapy will vary from company to company, but typically refers to very short-term therapy for concrete and uncomfortable symptoms. Once the immediate symptoms have improved, therapy is no longer covered. Preventative care is not a covered benefit.

This criteria has been used to disqualify most DSM-IV Axis II illnesses and some Axis I problems as well:

A client with a serious eating disorder had been working in therapy for approximately six sessions. While the managed care company had approved eight sessions with the option to call utilization review for more, the company sent notice that all approved sessions would have to be reapproved after January 1st of the new year. When the therapist called to do so, she was informed that as of January 1, anorexia nervosa was considered a "chronic" condition and not covered under the client's crisis managed care benefit.

A client who suffered from repeated bouts of serious depression was covered for crisis treatment of several discreet episodes of major depression as described in DSM-IV. Psychotherapy in between episodes was not covered. After several treatment episodes, the company refused to cover further treatment, saying the client was "chronically in crisis" and therefore not eligible for a crisis benefit.

Client misinformation about covered benefits

Few of the clients who come for therapy are aware of the limits of the treatment for mental health. The policy may simply say that the benefit includes a certain number (e.g., 20) of medically necessary outpatient sessions. Most clients assume this means they will receive 20 sessions if the therapist and client feel it is needed. It is important to clarify the limits to the client as soon as possible so that the client does not feel summarily abandoned or dismissed once therapy has begun.

The process of utilization review for a given company should also be reviewed early on since many clients are not aware of the limits of confidentiality and the tenuous nature of continuing therapy under some managed care companies. Upon signing the policy, managed care consumers usually have signed a release of information form allowing the company access to all information about the client's treatment. The release may have been buried in several pages of information and agreements, so the client may not remember or realize she has signed such a private release of information. Services will not be covered unless the information requested by the company is provided.

Another frequent unknown for the client is the role of utilization review in ongoing treatment. Most managed care companies require ongoing review of the inpatient or outpatient care. If the company requires frequent reviews (e.g., every two to four sessions), the client and therapist may not know from one session to the next if therapy may continue. It is best to inform clients of the potential for abrupt disruption of coverage and to plan an alternative should this happen.

The authors have thus far never had a course of psychotherapy discontinued on the spot without warning, but the potential remains. Typically, the reviewer gives some indication that ending this episode of covered therapy will likely happen soon or at the next utilization review. And clients may not realize that certain procedures such as psychological testing, custody evaluations, and fitness for duty evaluations are not covered by many companies. Check these procedures out with the company before they begin.

Make good-faith efforts to communicate

Communicating with managed care companies requires patience, civility, persistence, and assertiveness. Because these are the very skills needed to be an effective counselor, therapists should be well suited for these tasks. Mental health clients can be poorly equipped to deal with the complexity, frustration, and limits of their managed care company. In addition, most managed care companies require some sort of direct contact with the therapist.

As with most businesses, managed care companies have separate divisions for different company functions. The first task, then, is to determine which division to contact. Problems with unpaid bills will be handled by the claims departments, but questions about appropriate fees or client co-payments will be handled elsewhere. Client eligibility will likely be determined in a department separate from registration for treatment. It is useful to have phone numbers for all of these places. Waiting for a return call after leaving a message can waste valuable time, particularly if the wrong department has been contacted.

Written communication can also be effective if time is not an issue and the correct department and person is known. The advantage to written communication is that a record of the communication remains with the therapist:

> A therapist decided to resign from a managed care company and wrote to the director of the behavioral health department indicating her plan. Several months later she was still receiving referrals and provider literature from the company. This time she called to find out who should receive the resignation letter. She then wrote to the person indicated. When she still was listed as a member of the company's provider panel three months later, she felt comfortable ignoring it. She had documentation of her efforts to resign.

Utilization review

As practiced in managed mental health care, utilization review is the process by which the managed care company determines if the client's problems, the therapist's interventions, and the setting are covered benefits under the company's policy (Higuchi, 1994; Yenney, 1994). It can be as simple as requiring that the therapist provide information on diagnosis and procedure or a complex, 10-page form with data on all aspects of the client's life, history, and treatment (including detailed information on previous therapies and therapists).

Utilization review of individual clients usually is in the form of a written document that is periodically sent to the company or a telephone review with a reviewer. Paper reviews allow the therapist time to think about how to conceptualize and can be done during free hours. Disadvantages include risk of loss of confidentiality since the paper is sent in the mail, by fax, or by electronic means. Paper reviews also run the risk of becoming lost in the mail or at the company:

> A therapist completed the paper review for his client the required three weeks in advance of the last approved session and mailed it promptly. He continued to see his client in order to maintain the continuity of treatment and called after two weeks to see if a decision had been made. He was told the paper was "not in the system," but that the reviewers were running behind and it would likely be reviewed in the next few weeks. When five weeks had passed without word, he again called the company. He was informed that there was "no record"

of the review and the last few sessions he conducted would not be paid because he had not submitted a review. When he submitted a photocopy of the original, it was approved for sessions after the date that the photocopy was received. The sessions conducted in-between were not covered.

A therapist reported that a specific health plan was only authorizing one to two visits per utilization review for a client. Telephone reviews could only be scheduled two to three weeks in advance, requiring the client to frequently be seen without authorization. For the latest review the case manager called the wrong number and then took another call, again leaving the client without authorization.

A company managing the mental health benefits for a large health care company required that therapists call to schedule utilization review after a specified number of sessions. The therapists were required to leave a message on voicemail indicating three separate times that the managed care reviewer could call for utilization review. The company agreed to call back to confirm one of the times. However, the call was often not returned for several days. Meanwhile, therapists were required to keep those times open (all during business hours). Calls were frequently not returned at all, and eventually the company's voicemail was filled so that it was impossible even to leave a request for utilization review.

Telephone reviews have the potential to be helpful. The reviewer may have observations or questions that the therapist had not considered, much as a peer supervisor might. The therapist also has a chance to clarify misunderstandings with the reviewer before they result in rejection of further sessions. Finally, the therapist can get feedback on session approval at the time of the review rather than having to wait until written feedback arrives.

One of the most frustrating difficulties with telephone reviews is finding time to call. Few companies schedule these reviews at the therapist's convenience, but rather require the therapist to schedule an appointment with the reviewer; times are set by the company and rarely include evening or weekend hours. Some allow you to set a time that you wish as long as it does not interfere with the company's schedule. Others conduct their reviews at the time the call is made, but may keep the therapist on hold for as long as 30 minutes. Therapists tend to try to complete these reviews during lunch time or schedule a few free hours during the weekday.

One clinician reported that her temper is particularly strained when she has scheduled a review at the time designated by a managed care company and the reviewer is not available during the time designated. The clinician has scheduled free time and has a client waiting to learn the results of the review only to discover that the reviewer has not made him or herself available at the agreed-upon time. The review must then be rescheduled. Unfortunately, the clinician reports that this experience has occurred with multiple companies on multiple occasions.

A therapist indicated that two patients had received sessions approved during a December utilization review. However, the health plan would not allow those approved sessions to be forwarded to the following year. The therapist scheduled another utilization review, but the reviewer did not call at the scheduled time. The therapist called and was told the reviewer was running 45 minutes late. Because of another scheduled session, the therapist rescheduled the utilization review. One patient became fearful of scheduling sessions without authorization because of this and because the plan had not paid for previously authorized sessions.

The therapist should be prepared for the review. The same kind of information required in paper reviews will be required for telephone reviews. This will likely include demographic information, all five DSM-IV axes, clinical formulation, client history, signs and symptoms, and measurable, concrete, therapeutic goals and interventions. A company many also require other information specific to that company's policies. These reviews can be very pleasant or quite unpleasant. Preparing in advance as well as reviewing the company's clinical policies will minimize an unpleasant experience. However, if the therapist is prepared and still has a critical or negative response from the reviewer, the therapist needs to maintain perspective and keep a thick skin.

Treatment plans

As mentioned, treatment plans may be communicated via phone review with a managed care representative, paper review via completing the company's document, or the submission of written "supporting documentation." Occasionally a company will require that all progress notes be forwarded to the company for utilization review in addition to or instead of a formal treatment plan.

Many systems for constructing good treatment plans exist. All include a clinical formulation of the difficulties (e.g., diagnosis or a similar description of the client's reasons for pursuing counseling), a description of how the counselor plans to intervene, and an expected or desired outcome.

General instructions for designing good overall treatment plans are outside the scope of this book. We summarize, however, several guidelines for maximizing effective treatment plans for managed care.

For the purposes of this book, an effective treatment plan is one that is most likely to result in cooperation from the managed care company and allow the counselor to work competently. In addition to psychotherapeutic skill, knowledge of DSM-IV, and the medical model of mental health, the counselor will need an ability to describe client difficulties in behavioral terms. It is vital to have a detailed knowledge of each company's treatment and diagnostic requirements. Included in this should be a current knowledge of the company's diagnostic and treatment inclusions and exclusions. Note that they can change from month to month or from reviewer to reviewer.

Goodman et al. (1992) describe a treatment plan template that fits specific interventions to a specific behavioral impairment. They wisely point out that the commonly used terms "goals" and "objectives" lack clarity and consistency. Yet, utilization review will often require the clinician to describe treatment in these terms. It is generally best to be as specific and concrete as possible when constructing goals and objectives for a company:

> A therapist with a suicidal client described the goal to the reviewer as "the elimination of suicidal behaviors for at least six months." The objectives included having the client sign a contract not to engage in suicidal behaviors.

While the above vignette describes an "effective" treatment plan (i.e., the managed care company allowed the therapist to proceed with treatment), several discrepancies did exist between the written plan and its eventual implementation and outcome.

First, treatment was not allowed to continue past four months of weekly visits. The time frame outlined is not possible within the parameters of the allowable managed care treatment. Also, the process of having the client sign the contract is not described. Did the therapist convince the client that a contract was a good idea? Did the therapist coerce the client into signing it? Depending upon the process, the usefulness and strength of a signed, written suicide contract varies considerably.

Obviously, the treatment plan described to a utilization reviewer cannot substitute for the comprehensive, complex, and Socratic nature of the therapeutic relationship. Nor does an accepted treatment plan release the counselor from the detailed conceptual work necessary to work well with a client. These things must happen *in addition* to a successful utilization review.

General communication skills

Regardless of the type of communication with the managed care company, a few basic principles are worth remembering. Familiarize yourself with the specific procedures of each company before you contact them. One company may rarely call back when voicemail is left, but responds in person if the call is made early in the morning. Another company may require that communication be by fax rather than by e-mail. Colleagues are an excellent source of information about the specifics of various companies.

Remain polite, no matter how rude or frustrating the response from the company. Angry letters written to company officers rarely get a response. Sarcastic comments to utilization reviewers may jeopardize the number of sessions your client receives. Criticizing claims personnel will delay, rather than speed the correct processing of the billing error.

On the other hand, be direct and firm. Request to speak to a supervisor if an issue is not resolved to your satisfaction. Particularly with regard to client needs, it is important to advocate as strongly as is necessary to be effective. Persistence can also help further a goal. Calling back to speak to another company representative may be as effective as pushing repeatedly with the same person. Most companies have some staff that are genuinely interested in resolving difficulties.

Finally, cultivate relationships with company personnel if possible. Utilization reviewers often develop opinions about the clinicians they review. If the counselor is always annoyed, demeaning, or pushing the limits of session numbers, he or she may develop a reputation that will decrease overall effectiveness. The clinician that uses his or her best therapeutic skills with company representatives will maximize the ability to provide therapy to the client for whom he or she is calling.

Summary

One overall effect of many of the rules, procedures, and processes of managed mental health care is to discourage the use of counseling services. In the name of quality and cost control, companies place obstacles in the way of both clients and counselors. Clients must deal with delays in seeing counselors, less choice about who they see, limits on the number of sessions, and higher costs for counseling (as compared to medical) services. Counselors and counseling agencies must cope with restricted provider panels, extensive application materials and contracts, intrusive and frequent utilization reviews, delayed payments, and greater administrative expenses and effort. In spite of this, skilled counselors and motivated clients can still find ways to connect and collaborate.

Managed Care and the Counseling Process

While the introduction of managed care has revolutionized the manner in which mental health services are delivered, nowhere are the changes more noticeable than in the therapy room. Many basic assumptions about how psychotherapy should proceed are no longer feasible in the current managed care environment. Counselors may need to change the fundamentals of how they counsel or decide to operate outside the managed care system.

This chapter describes the counseling process and the decisions a counselor may need to make to provide the best therapy in a managed care setting. These differences are possible regardless of the therapist's work setting, be it agency, clinic, school, hospital, managed care company, or private practice. Some changes have the potential to improve the counseling process if handled properly, and some will not improve or harm the process.

Some changes introduced by managed care are clearly detrimental, so that decisions become more difficult. Does the counselor act to minimize the harm as much as possible? Or, are some changes so significant that the counselor cannot practice competently within the context of the managed care requirements? Flexibility, creativity, and self-awareness are the tools most necessary to the counselor as she or he negotiates this area.

Changes in the initial session

A plethora of theories exist regarding how to structure the first session between counselor and client (Adams, Piercy, & Jurich, 1991; Gunzburger, Henggeler, & Watson, 1985; Odell & Quinn, 1998). Some theorists recommend an open-ended, nondirectional approach to meeting with the client for the first time. This approach allows the client to tell his or her story in his or her own way. The therapist can gain important information in this way: What does the client consider the most important elements of his or her situation? How does the client understand what is going on in his or her life? What does the client feel the structure of therapy should be? What does the client leave unsaid?

Typically, this sort of initial session begins with a nondirectional invitation to talk such as, "Tell me what I might help you with" or "What brings you to therapy today?" In addition to providing vital information about the client's way of organizing his or her experience and difficulties, this approach also can help establish a working alliance early on (Meier & Davis, 2000). The client feels able to talk to someone who is listening closely without interrupting. Other theorists believe that, at minimum, the initial session should be structured so that important and relevant areas are not missed (cf. Lubin, Loris, Burt, & Johnson, 1998; Sommers-Flanagan & Sommers-Flanagan, 1999). A client who does not volunteer her drinking problem when allowed simply to talk may not get the immediate and necessary help she needs to benefit from psychotherapy. Likewise, it may be critical to ascertain the presence of suicidal thoughts and plans to prevent a death.

Given that many other sources describe what to cover in an initial structured interview, this chapter will focus on the type of material one must address to meet the requirements of many managed care utilization reviews.

Few managed care companies allocate unlimited therapy sessions without requiring utilization review. However, the companies vary widely with regard to the number of sessions the counselor may conduct prior to a review. Some companies require the client to call a triage caseworker for the company and describe the symptoms before an initial session will be authorized.

> One client called her managed care company and described some mild depression and difficulty deciding on a career. The managed care worker told her that unless she was "ready to jump off a bridge or something" she was not covered by her insurance for psychotherapy. The client opted to see a therapist anyway and paid for the therapy herself.

Some companies allocate one or two initial evaluation sessions for the purpose of gathering information and designing a treatment plan. In this case, the therapist must gather all of the data required for utilization review in the first one or two sessions. While the information varies from company to company (in fact, no two companies seem to require quite the same information), some categories appear almost universal.

The medical model

Most utilization reviews rely heavily on the medical model approach to mental health. This means that, at minimum, the counselor will need to be familiar with and able to diagnose his or her client using all five axes of the DSM-IV (Diagnostic & Statistical Manual, American Psychiatric Association, 1994):

- Axis I, Major Psychiatric Disorders, including Anorexia Nervosa and Major Depression: This axis includes all the DSM-IV disorders except personality disorders and mental retardation.
- Axis II, Personality Disorders, including Borderline Personality Disorder: This axis is used to report personality disorders and mental retardation.
- Axis III, General Medical Disorders: Medical conditions that may be relevant to a mental disorder are listed on this axis.
- Axis IV, Psychosocial and Environmental Factors: Any psychosocial or environmental condition that could affect the mental disorders should be described on this axis.
- Axis V, Global Functioning: This axis is used to record the counselor's assessment of the overall level of the functioning of the client. The most commonly used measure, the Global Assessment of Functioning Scale (Endicott, Spitzer, Fleiss, and Cohen, 1976) rates psychological, social, and occupational functioning on a 1–100-point scale.

Symptom description

Therapists should be prepared to describe the symptoms the client is experiencing. Again, the medical model prevails, so difficulties such as existential anxiety, feeling stuck, loneliness, or career indecision may not be accepted. The DSM-IV is a useful guide to the types of symptoms considered in a managed care setting.

A therapist was working with an impulsive client who had difficulty making constructive decisions, particularly with her children. When the therapist described this difficulty to the managed care reviewer, she was informed that the HMO does not cover parenting skills.

Risk

Therapists should know if the client is suicidal, homicidal, or has been so in the past (Sommers-Flanagan & Sommers-Flanagan, 1999). The therapist may be asked if the client has a suicide or homicide plan and/or the means to carry it out. The therapist may be asked to rate the estimated level of lethality and if the client agreed to some sort of contract not to act on the suicidal or homicidal thoughts.

Drugs and alcohol

The client's drug and alcohol use or abuse is frequently questioned (Sommers-Flanagan & Sommers-Flanagan, 1999). If the client does abuse these substances, the managed care reviewer may require that the client undergo a drug and alcohol evaluation and/or treatment prior to or instead of psychotherapy. Unless the therapist meets company criteria for drug and alcohol treatment (usually a Certified Alcohol Counselor credential, regardless of the therapist's degree or training), this phase must happen at one of the company's approved drug and alcohol sites. The rigid application of this alcohol treatment criterion can sometimes be problematic:

> A client with a serious eating disorder phoned her managed care company to receive approval to see a therapist skilled in treating eating disorders. As part of the routine, the managed care worker asked her if she ever became drunk after using alcohol. The client replied that occasionally she did drink too much when she was out with friends. On the basis of that answer, the client was prohibited from seeing the therapist until she underwent an evaluation for alcohol abuse. The evaluation determined that she did not need treatment for alcohol abuse and she was approved for psychotherapy for her eating disorder. However, five weeks had passed while the evaluation was scheduled and conducted. During that time the client was binging and purging three to four times a day.

Psychosocial and mental health history

HMO reviewers vary widely regarding how much historical information they require about a client (Sommers-Flanagan & Sommers-Flanagan, 1999). Some ask only a few questions, and others require very extensive data about the client's past.

Many will want to know about past episodes of mental health difficulties, particularly episodes similar to the current problems. Because problems that have happened repeatedly or have been troubling the client for some time have the danger of being labeled "chronic" by the reviewer, this can be a tricky issue for the therapist. If the HMO covers only "acute" mental health problems, the length of the problem can be used as a criterion to exclude the client from coverage. Likewise, if the therapist has been seeing the client for therapy and the client changes insurance coverage, the reviewer for the new insurance may decide that the client has used up his or her "acute" benefit under the previous policy.

A therapist called the managed care reviewer to request further sessions for a suicidal client. The reviewer had been informed that this particular client had been in a mental health crisis many times before. The reviewer decided that the client's current symptoms did constitute a crisis, but that the client was "chronically in crisis" and not eligible for further benefits.

Other areas that are frequently questioned are:

- family members with current or past mental health problems,
- current or past legal trouble,
- history of child abuse,
- previous medical illnesses,
- domestic violence, and
- educational/academic history.

Medications

Therapists will almost always be asked about the client's medications, both psychotropic and medical (Sommers-Flanagan & Sommers-Flanagan, 1999). Therapists may also be asked about the dosage levels of these medications and the name(s) of prescribing physicians. Sometimes the last date of contact between the client and the prescribing physician is required (despite the fact that this information is probably available to the reviewer if the physician submitted a claim to the client's company for his or her services).

Finally, the therapist may be asked when he or she last contacted the physician on the client's behalf. Many HMOs consider close contact between all providers of health services and physicians a crucial part of comprehensive health care. There are some real advantages to this model. Many mental health concerns can influence physical health. The converse is also true. If all health care givers are in contact, coordination of services can be maximized to the client's benefit. However, some clients view their mental health concerns as embarrassing and are reluctant to share needed information with the therapist if it may find its way to the primary care physician.

Mental status exam

Some companies require very formal mental status examinations and some require only bits and pieces of a mental status exam (Sommers-Flanagan &

Sommers-Flanagan, 1999). This exam is not standardized, but many examples of the usually required data and assessment tool exist (e.g., Wiger, 1999). Again, this is a structured interview technique often associated with the psychiatric/medical model.

If a formal mental status exam is not required, it may be possible to provide the HMO with the required information based on the first session interview itself:

> An HMO required that the therapist provide information after the first session about the client's orientation to person, place, and time (a standard mental status exam question). During the interview, the client had accurately described himself coming to the therapist's office on the correct day and time. On the basis of this, the therapist was able to tell the HMO that the client was "oriented x3."

Role induction

An important part of most first sessions is the opportunity to educate clients about the function and process of therapy. This is typically referred to as role induction and thorough descriptions can be found elsewhere (cf. Meier & Davis, 1990). Adding information regarding the client's managed care company policies is strongly recommended because they have such an important impact on the direction the therapy may take. However, including this information in a sensitive and professional manner can be difficult, particularly if the client is distraught or in crisis.

If the client must preregister with the company, the therapist will need to ascertain if this has happened prior to meeting with the client. Therapists may be required to collect referral slips from Primary Care Physicians (PCPs) or copayments in a first session. Often clients are not aware that their copayment for mental health may be different from what they are used to paying for a medical office visit. Some psychotherapy copays are as large as 50 percent of the fee. A client who is already upset may find it quite stressful to find she or he owes $40 to $50 for each visit. Sometimes the copays start out at a smaller fee (e.g., $5 to $15) and then increase after several visits. Clients should be prepared for these changes.

It is not enough to simply ask the client if he or she has reviewed the HMO policy for mental health. Often the literature is difficult to understand and may not state explicitly the practical limits of coverage.

> A client came for a first session with a therapist and disclosed that the company representative told him he would have up to 20 sessions as long as the therapist felt they were necessary. In fact, the therapist did feel they would be necessary, but the managed care reviewer limited

the number covered to 12, stating, "We almost never give all 20 for that diagnosis." The client called the company back and was again told he would receive all 20 if "medically necessary." The client was caught between the therapist and the company and could not tell whom to believe.

In practice, it is recommended that the therapist talk openly with the client about the actual limits of coverage for that company. If a particular HMO typically approves 6 to 12 sessions for a given diagnosis, but the therapist suspects the therapy will take longer, it is important to share this information with the client so that he or she can make an informed decision about how to proceed. For example, a therapist may say:

> I know your HMO policy states that you have coverage for up to 20 sessions if they are medically necessary, but in my experience with this company, they typically allow only 10 as medically necessary for your diagnosis. I do not know how many they will actually approve for you. That will be based in part on how well I am able to make a case for more sessions with the HMO reviewer. However, there is a chance that you will run out of covered sessions before we both feel you are finished. I want to let you know about this at the beginning so that you can make an informed choice about therapy.

> I see several options. First, you may be able pay for sessions on your own if they are not covered by the HMO. You may also wish to look for a therapist who feels she or he can finish with you in the time covered by the insurance. I can refer you to a mental health agency that may use a sliding scale fee to calculate what you will owe if you pay on your own. Finally, you can postpone therapy if you feel able to wait.

Many therapists decide to reduce fees for clients who cannot afford to continue. The difficulty here is that it may be considered fraudulent to bill an insurance company one fee and then bill a lesser fee to the client for the same service (Sands, Cullen, & Higuchi, 1996). Thus, the therapist cannot legally charge full price while insurance is being used and then switch to a lower fee when the client is paying on his or own. Since all insurance billing for the same service must be at the same fee, a particular client's insurance cannot be billed at a reduced fee in anticipation that the client will continue at that fee once further sessions have been denied by the HMO.

Confidentiality

Confidentiality is another potentially important area to cover as part of managed care role induction. When signing up for coverage, most managed care companies require the client to sign a release of information form for the company. Clients may not remember having signed such a release or may not think it applies to mental health issues. Clients should be informed that specific information about private matters as they pertain to the therapy may be requested by the company. Clients do have the right to refuse disclosure, but run the risk that the company will not cover the therapy.

We often show our clients a copy of the form the company requires the therapist to complete to request therapy sessions. The client then knows what information will need to be disclosed for the sessions to be covered by the HMO.

While maintaining confidentiality has always been a cornerstone of counseling and psychotherapy, for some managed care companies it is unfamiliar terrain. Most practitioners have one or more experiences of the following sort:

A therapist received a letter from a health plan reviewing treatment of five patients with depressive disorder, with their subscriber numbers attached. None of the individuals were the therapist's patients. When he called the health plan, they indicated that such letters (with the wrong patients per provider) had been sent to all providers.

A counselor receives a request from a plan to submit a copy of two patient records for a "research project on depression." His secretary hand delivers the materials to the company. The next week a representative of the plan telephones and asks where the records are. After explaining they were delivered the previous week, the company does find them. The following week another representative from the plan calls and asks for the same records. When told they had been delivered two weeks ago, this person asks to whom and what department they had been delivered.

Balancing the client's needs with the therapist and the HMO

In the current climate, few managed care clients come to therapy without pressing issues. The initial session may be the first time the client has met with a therapist, the client may be uncertain about the benefits of therapy, the client may be fearful of the therapist, or the client may be very upset and wanting immediate relief. Whatever the case, there is often very little time to cover the information required by all the parties, establish rapport, and provide a hopeful, empathic environment.

One strategy is to deal with client issues first and save time during the next few sessions to deal with the managed care limits and requirements.

In the same way, some therapists say little about the managed care review process if they feel the company is likely to approve some treatment. Hopefully, by the time the company begins to limit sessions, the client will be out of crisis and better able to problem solve. At that time the client can choose to continue by paying for therapy her- or himself or can terminate with the benefits of the work accomplished so far. If the managed care company is reasonable about its utilization policy, the therapist, client, and company can agree that it is time to end therapy.

Potential problems, however, exist with this approach. Often the therapist, client, and managed care company do not agree that therapy should end at a certain point. If the therapist and client agree that more sessions are indicated but the company does not agree, the client may not understand why she or he is being terminated so unexpectedly. Also, the client has not had the opportunity to explore other options for help with the limited sessions she does have available.

Another approach is to provide all clients with information about requirements and limits prior to the first session. This can be accomplished by mailing information sheets to clients or giving them to the client in the office before the session begins. The therapist could also have office staff explain the benefits or call the client prior to the session and explain. Finally, some therapists feel that the benefits and limits of coverage are the responsibility of the client and do not deal with them at all in therapy. The therapist may simply tell the client to consult the company for further information.

Each of these approaches has the potential for positive and negative effects. While it is important to hold the client responsible for the therapy, many clients have genuine difficulty deciphering their policy limits. The conclusions drawn by reading the benefits manual or calling a customer representative may be different from the way the limits are enforced in practice. The client feels surprised and betrayed when the policy limits reached are discrepant from the ones outlined by the customer representative or manual. Likewise, providing information about the limits of therapy and extensive information about the copay and costs involved can be discouraging to a client who is reluctant to start therapy or wonders if the therapist will be empathic and understanding.

Saving the discussion of money and policy limits until the end of the first session runs the risk that the therapist may not be comfortable switching topics from issues to money quickly enough to allow the time necessary to discuss it. It may be very difficult for a client to understand the therapist's need to do this when his or her presenting issues are so painful and unfinished.

Whichever method or combination of methods the therapist decides to use, the key is to approach the topic with sensitivity and openness. It is easy to become defensive when the client is accusing you of caring more about money than him. It is also easy to shift all the heat to the managed care company and adopt a "what can I do?" stance. It is paramount that the therapist resists these understandable inclinations and listens to how the client reacts to the information provided. After all, even this is grist for the mill. Balancing the need to gather utilization review information, provide information about limits and copays, and listen well to the client's story, all within the first 50 to 60 minutes of meeting the client, is an exquisitely difficult task. Some feel it is impossible.

The process of therapy

Regardless of theoretical orientation, traditional therapeutic approaches rarely include an exact number of therapy sessions. Even highly structured behavioral interventions rarely specify the exact number of sessions in the initial evaluation. Rather, the decision is made as therapy progresses and treatment gains are observed by therapist and client.

Some exceptions exist to this model. Closed groups often meet for a specified number of times. College counseling centers have long limited the length of therapy to the length of the semester (often with the stipulation that therapy could resume the next semester or the client could be referred to a longer-term therapist). Currently, a number of empirically validated treatment protocols use group or individual sessions in a very structured format (e.g., Zinbarg, Craske, & Barlow, 1993).

Deciding on therapy goals and estimating the number of sessions required to reach the goals is an uncertain project. Little data exists on the average number of sessions needed to achieve a particular therapeutic goal (cf. Howard, Kopta, Krause, & Orlinsky, 1986; Kadera, Lambert, & Andrews, 1996). The speed with which a person changes varies as a result of a number of variables, including the difficulty of the goal, motivation to change, experience and expertise of the therapist, amount of intra-session practice, amount of psychopathology that interferes with change, and how conducive the environment is to change.

Many managed care companies require the therapist to estimate the number of sessions needed. Based on the data the therapist provides and the company's decision-making protocols, a number is assigned. Some companies appear to assign the same number of sessions regardless of the diagnosis or treatment goals. This practice places the therapist in an unanticipated situation in which treatment goals must be generated based on the number assigned by the company rather than the other way around. The therapist should discuss this with the client and try to outline what can and cannot be accomplished in the time allocated. Sometimes treatment goals must be prioritized because they all cannot be reached. The client should have some say about which goals should come first. Some treatment goals simply cannot be accomplished with the number of sessions allocated.

If the managed care company refuses additional sessions, clients and therapists react in several ways. Clients commonly react by feeling that either they or their therapist have somehow failed. If the managed care company indicates that enough sessions have been allocated, some clients fear that they have just not worked hard enough or are just too "sick" to have responded well. Other clients feel hurt and angry that the therapist did not try hard enough or did not advocate strongly enough for them with the managed care company. The therapist must inquire about these feelings as the therapy progresses and when the session limits are finished:

> A client with a serious eating disorder and perfectionistic expectations of herself was given a total of 12 sessions to resolve these problems. When the 12 were up, the client had made some progress, but still needed more therapy to solidify gains and manage her eating. Her parents had unreasonably high expectations for their daughter and expected her to resolve her difficulties quickly. They couldn't understand why she didn't "just eat." When the insurance refused to authorize more sessions, the daughter was afraid to tell her parents. She feared she would fail once again in their eyes. As a result she was not able to ask them for financial help with continuing therapy.

Therapy style and limited sessions

Limiting the number of sessions has had a profound effect on the ways in which therapy is typically practiced. This section will describe some of the changes and the decisions that must be made. Therapists often have been taught the theory and practice of psychotherapy in an environment that does not limit the length of therapy. A notable exception to this observation is the number of brief therapy training courses now taught as continuing education and in graduate programs (e.g., Budman, 1983; Budman & Gurman, 1996; Cummings, Budman, & Thomas, 1998; Lopez, 1985). Even within a brief therapy model, the average number of sessions recommended for a satisfactory outcome may be greater than the number allocated by some managed care companies.

Most theoretical orientations do not specify a length of treatment, but many are commonly classified as short term or long term. This distinction may be useful as a broad classification, but still does not specify the exact length of therapy. Therefore, a cognitive-behavioral approach to a complex personality disorder may take some time, even though cognitive-behavioral interventions often are seen as short-term interventions, whereas a psychoanalytic treatment of a single episode, mild depression in an insightful client may not take very long at all.

Supposedly, the number of sessions granted by the utilization reviewer is based on the specifics of the clinical picture as presented by the therapist or through some other assessment tool (e.g., scores on a measure of symptoms or functioning). Therapy proceeds through each goal and is periodically reviewed as sessions are used. In practice, the number of sessions granted can seem to have little to do with the client's particular situation:

> Several therapists noticed that no matter what the presenting complaint of the client or how distressed the client seemed to be, the managed care company always granted four sessions at a time with a requirement that the utilization process should be repeated if more sessions were needed. This always occurred after a full 15 to 20-minute review over the phone with the managed care reviewer.

Another company did vary the number granted (usually between two and six) based on the DSM-IV Axis I diagnosis given. Even though the severity of the symptoms or situation varied from client to client, and despite the requirement that an extensive three-page form be completed each time, the number of sessions remained constant.

Therapy goals

When the number of sessions is uncertain or too small, the therapist and client must alter the way they design therapeutic goals. One can limit the goals to the most distressing current symptoms and agree to address contributing or less distressing issues at another time. Cummings and Sayama (1995), for example, have described a model of psychotherapy that allows clients throughout the life cycle to return to therapy periodically for short-term interventions when issues or symptoms become distressing.

If the amount of time necessary to make the changes desired by the client is likely not enough, the therapist must make a choice. Among the counselor's choices are to:

- share this view with the client so that both can decide about proceeding as far as they can,
- help clients consider whether to pay for therapy when sessions are used up,
- refer the client to a counseling agency with the ability to continue therapy post insurance.

If the final option is chosen, it is important that the therapist refer the client immediately. Using up clients' insurance benefits and then sending them to an agency is both unethical and counter-therapeutic. In addition, some agencies are no longer able to afford continued therapy once the HMO has refused further sessions. Of course, the therapist may also decide to continue the client pro bono or at a significantly reduced fee.

An additional possibility is to present a positive and hopeful approach to the time allowed. The therapist can admit that the time may not be enough, but expect the client will obtain significant relief if both client and therapist focus and work together. Instilling hope is an important part of the therapeutic process (Frank, 1971). Clients can humble therapists who expect too little of them:

> A therapist was impressed when a client struggling with agoraphobia with panic improved significantly after four sessions. The client had already completed a group therapy with little relief and had been suffering for the past year. The client used the session limits as an incentive to confront her fears consistently and forcefully between sessions. At termination, the client still had some difficulties, but was comfortable enough to resume most activities. In addition, she felt she had the tools to continue to improve.

Preaching

When time is limited, clinicians must resist the impulse to preach. Psychoeducation may constitute a valuable part of counseling, but should not be confused with throwing out as much information as one can in a limited time (Meier & Davis, 1990). Some therapists hope that the client can digest and make use of a large amount of information. Other therapists have difficulty sorting through and prioritizing the information relevant to a given client. Likewise, some therapists feel a need to frantically correct as many of the client's cognitive and behavioral mistakes as possible. Finally, some therapists need to make and deliver as many interpretations of maladaptive behavior as possible, regardless of whether or not the client is ready for them.

In addition to pushing themselves too hard, therapists may find themselves pushing clients to change more rapidly than they are able. Pushing oneself and/or the client faster than is reasonable rarely leads to a positive outcome (Meier & Davis, 1990). Therapists can find themselves frustrated with themselves and their clients. Clients are vulnerable to fears of disappointing the therapist or feeling as though they have failed at yet another task. It is better to end therapy with a mildly improved client than to risk turning therapy into a negative experience to be avoided in the future.

Exaggerating the diagnosis or symptoms

A therapist may be tempted to exaggerate her client's symptoms to the utilization reviewer in order to gain extra time to work. If the number of sessions granted is too small (as it often is), one can make the case that the client's best interest is served by doing what is necessary to obtain adequate care. Some clients may not strictly meet criteria for a medically necessary DSM-IV diagnosis, yet clearly need counseling.

The negative effects on the therapeutic relationship must be considered and weighed, however. If the therapist is not honest with the utilization reviewer, how can she feel comfortable presenting therapy as an open and honest place to explore oneself? If the therapist is honest with the client about exaggerating symptoms, the therapy can be set up as a place in which the "good children" are plotting against the "big, bad company." The message sent by either of these strategies is clearly counter-therapeutic. Finally, the therapist is violating the terms of the contract she signed with the company and perhaps committing insurance fraud.

Session frequency

Traditionally, therapy sessions were scheduled for a minimum of once per week. The rationale, in part, held that weekly sessions gave clients enough time in between sessions to work on changing, but were frequent enough to reduce avoidance of critical issues. A therapist could keep the client's life situation and issues in awareness more easily if a week or less went by between sessions. If a client was in crisis, the weekly session was usually the minimum needed to monitor the client's status.

Managed care has significantly changed how therapists and clients think about the frequency of sessions (Cummings & Sayama, 1995). Some managed care companies actively discourage weekly sessions in favor of bimonthly or monthly visits. A therapist must provide a client-specific rationale if she wishes to see a client weekly or more frequently. Others allow clients to start weekly, but quickly push to have the frequency reduced.

A therapist worked with a managed care client with a serious schizoaffective disorder. The client did well in once-weekly outpatient psychotherapy for some time, but began to seriously decompensate when her divorce became final. Although this client had a history of serious suicide attempts, became psychotic often, and required frequent hospitalizations, the HMO refused to allow the client to continue seeing the therapist weekly because the weekly sessions had been going on for "too long." When the therapist suggested that reducing the frequency of sessions could result in even more hospitalizations and greater cost to the HMO, he was told that "the inpatient treatment is another department and has a separate budget that does not affect us."

At other times, the HMO does not specify the frequency of treatment sessions, but simply limits the overall number. In those cases the therapist must choose between a short, intense treatment period or a longer, less intense plan. The needs of the client should dictate this decision. Some clients with relatively acute circumscribed problems may respond rapidly and well to a short, intense therapy. Clients with more diverse, chronic, and pervasive issues may be best served by stretching out sessions at low frequency for as long as possible. In either case, the rationale should be shared with the client.

Uncertain termination

Before managed care, the timing of termination was considered to be largely a decision between therapist and client. As such, the termination phase of treatment was an integral part of the treatment (Hill & O'Brien, 1999). A commonly held therapeutic precept stated that termination began with the initial interview (Meier & Davis, 1990). The process of terminating well was, in itself, a therapeutic goal designed to help the client work through unfinished issues of separation, abandonment, and self-reliance.

With its emphasis on ongoing utilization review, managed care has introduced a new wrinkle in the termination process. As described, ongoing utilization review usually requires that the therapist and/or client justify the need, utility, and cost-effectiveness of sessions beyond those authorized so far. Each new contact with utilization review carries the possibility of rejection of further sessions. Reviewers clearly vary in the quality of their decisions:

> A client with a history of severe sexual abuse by her father is very suicidal over the course of therapy, including at least one suicide attempt. Her managed care company proposes cutting her weekly sessions to biweekly. Her therapist convinces the company to extend weekly treatment by using the report of a psychiatric consultant and her elevated Beck Depression Inventory score. The plan agrees to two more months of weekly sessions, but indicates that counseling will be biweekly after that because "weekly sessions foster the patient's over-reliance on the therapist."

Therapists have a choice. They can (and are encouraged to do so by the HMO) set a termination time with the client. In this way, both client and therapist are motivated to use time efficiently with a strong focus on meeting the therapeutic goal. Additionally, some theorists have suggested that terminating at a specified time regardless of having completely met the goals can provide useful practice with transferring responsibility for change from therapist to client (cf. Budman, 1983). As long as the HMO allows for a reasonable time frame for meeting goals, this method may meet the client's needs. Often, however, the termination time cannot be set because utilization review is an ongoing process that does not allow the therapist to specify with certainty the length of treatment.

Despite the request that the therapist estimate length of treatment, many HMOs prefer to authorize sessions in small blocks with required utilization review after the sessions are used and before more are granted. The rationale is that the therapist and client have nothing to worry about if the client continues to have a medically necessary diagnosis and the therapy is progressing. More sessions will be granted.

In practice, the total number of sessions authorized is far fewer than many therapists find useful. The therapist cannot set a length of treatment goal with the client because it is uncertain and may be less than therapist and client agree is necessary. When therapist and client do not know when therapy will end, but are aware that it may be premature, the tone of the therapy changes significantly. Both therapist and client may be tempted to avoid connecting deeply. Exploring the transference becomes more difficult and less important as the focus shifts to implementing change quickly. The therapy can come to resemble the "expert-patient" model that is common in medicine:

> A therapist with a heavy managed care practice described the changes in her practice. She saw most of her clients once every two to three weeks for a couple of months. She had some difficulty remembering their names and made sure she reviewed them at the start of each day. She saw many clients for only three or four sessions. Even if the HMO approved more, many clients dropped out after only a few. She kept more extensive clinical notes, both to meet HMO requirements and to help her remember what was happening in her clients' lives. She could no longer trust her memory.

The therapist must decide how informed he or she wishes to keep clients about the tenuous nature of ongoing sessions. If the therapist does not inform the client in the hope that enough sessions are granted to finish, the client may be able to focus and connect more quickly and easily. The client is saved unnecessary worry and therapy time is not spent on this issue. In this scenario, the therapist balances the positives of not troubling the client with the negatives of a surprise termination (perhaps a greater detriment to the therapy). The therapist can also simply continue the therapy pro bono after session denial, but then must deal with his or her own feelings about not being paid.

An existential approach to the uncertainty may assist the therapist (Morse, 1998). Uncertainty about the future is an integral part of life and often a difficult concept for clients (and therapists) to accept. How does one live a happy life knowing that death may come suddenly at any time? How does one connect deeply with another person if that person may be gone without warning? These issues are important ones and can be worked through in the context of an uncertain therapy. The therapist must first be able to accept uncertainty to be able to use it in a productive way with a client.

Copayments

Some clients come to therapy expecting the co-payment for psychotherapy to be the same nominal amount that they pay for an office visit to a physician. They are unpleasantly surprised to learn that the counseling co-pay is often much more. Some clients cannot afford the co-pay and some are simply upset that therapy is so expensive. Therapists can become the target for anger over an issue they cannot control.

Dealing with a client who is angry at the therapist rather than the real target should be a familiar place for the therapist. It can be dealt with in the same way that the therapist would deal with any misdirected anger. The therapist must resist the impulse to become defensive and help the client clarify the issues and her or his feelings. As discussed in Chapter 2, the therapist may wish to make an effort to inform the client of the co-pay structure prior to the first session.

Termination

It should be clear by now that the HMO may deny payment for further sessions before client and therapist feel finished. Assuming the client cannot or will not pay for further work, and assuming the therapist cannot or will not reduce or eliminate the fee, termination will feel premature. As described, it is important that the therapist work through his or her feelings about this situation so that he or she is emotionally present and can non-defensively help the client with his or her thoughts and feelings. The client may blame herself for failing to meet an authority's (the HMO) goals, or she may blame the therapist. The client may feel abandoned by the therapist. After all, if the therapist really cared, wouldn't he see her for as long as needed?

In reality, the therapist does have an ethical and legal obligation to continue needed therapy regardless of payment status (Parvin & Anderson,

1995). If the therapist genuinely feels that the client is at risk without continued therapy and cannot find a suitable referral, she must continue with the client until the client is no longer at risk. Making a therapeutically sound and objective judgment can be difficult. The therapist must sort through the thoughts and feelings that arise in this situation, particularly if it happens frequently. The therapist may feel angry, resentful, used, and defiant. On the other hand, the therapist may have rescuing fantasies that pull for the client to be grateful. Therapists may particularly benefit in such instances from supervision or consultation with a colleague.

Insurance countertransference

Throughout this chapter the authors have attempted to describe some of the more common reactions of managed care clients in therapy. Therapist reactions and the responses to those reactions have also been covered. Self-awareness is critically important. Beginning therapists and those who have not encountered managed care will need to spend time examining their reactions to these new clinical situations.

Insurance countertransference describes the tendency to view clients with different managed care plans differently. All of the therapists' reactions described previously will vary depending on the specific policies of the client's managed care company. One company may make utilization review burdensome for the therapist while another routinely grants only a few sessions regardless of diagnosis. Still another pays the therapist a very low fee or frequently finds excuses for not paying at all.

> A clinician worked for several years with a managed care company that suddenly reduced its payment fee by one-fourth. She noticed that her interest in starting with new clients from this managed care plan had also declined. While she found the clients interesting and enjoyable to work with, she was distressed by her change in mood. She sought supervision from a colleague to help sort through these feelings.

A danger exists that a new hierarchy of psychotherapy will develop with the most skilled therapists unavailable to those with managed care coverage that is not clinician friendly. Therapists are challenged to examine basic beliefs about what matters to them as they practice. Money does matter to counselors, whether they receive a fee for a service or a salary as an employee. In our experience, however, good therapists always rank money at least one level below concern for the client. The ongoing self-evaluation that is so necessary to become and remain a good therapist should now include the feelings engendered by dealing with managed care.

Summary

Managed care can strongly influence the counseling process. With the constraints introduced by managed care, counselors often have less time to gather client information, establish rapport, and intervene in a therapeutic manner. The counselor may need to explain HMO policies and limits to clients and how they will affect the process, type, and length of therapy. Counseling may also be affected by how assertively and diplomatically the counselor can intervene with representatives of the managed care company. Thus, how the counselor handles the pressures and changes resulting from managed care can significantly help or hinder the counseling process and subsequent outcomes.

Outcome Assessment and Evaluation in Managed Care

One of the most valid criticisms that managed care companies (and the general public) may levy against counseling concerns the lack of information about quality and outcomes (Davis, 1998). As discussed in this chapter, we have fairly good evidence about the general effectiveness of psychotherapy, but far less certainty about the results of counseling with any particular client or group of clients. Theory and research about how to measure outcomes and evaluate quality remain relatively primitive.

Given the types and quantity of data they routinely collect, managed care companies have potentially important contributions to make to counseling and psychotherapy research. For example, many companies ask counselors and/or clients to provide outcome assessments, methods designed to gauge the level of therapeutic progress. Collected with hundreds or thousands of cases per problem area, these data have the potential to inform researchers and counselors about a variety of process and outcome questions. For example, while much data support the use of particular counseling approaches with specific problems such as depression or anxiety (i.e., empirically validated treatments, or EVTs), few studies have examined the effectiveness of such approaches with different ethnic minority groups (cf. Sue, 1999).

Do counseling and psychotherapy work?

One of the arguments employed by managed care companies to justify a decrease in mental health services is that a lack of evidence exists to support the effectiveness of counseling and psychotherapy. Kessler (1998), for example, maintained that employers have found that behavioral health care costs per members were higher than other areas, yet little data were available to demonstrate the effectiveness of those services. This combination meant that "there was little to stop payers from demanding ever-greater savings" (Kessler, 1998, p. 157). Kessler (1998, p. 159) sees no change coming here: "As we try to defend behavioral health's legitimate claim in an era of scarce resources, we have impaired credibility and little clout at the bargaining table."

But the argument that counseling lacks evidence of effectiveness is simply unfounded: hundreds of studies conducted since the 1950s document its general effectiveness (e.g., Bergin & Garfield, 1994; Meyer et al., 1998; Smith, Glass, & Miller, 1980; Sexton, Whiston, Bleuer, & Walz, 1997). Traditional and meta-analytic reviews of the literature consistently reach one conclusion: persons who complete counseling and psychotherapy have better outcomes than persons who do not.

Despite the clarity of this conclusion, once one moves into more complicated questions, the answers become considerably less conclusive. For example, one fundamental question pertinent to managed care is whether outcome is related to the number of sessions a client receives. In other words, is brief therapy as effective as long-term therapy? Here there are conflicting results. A recent *Consumer Reports* survey ("Does Therapy Help?", November 1995) of 4,000 readers who had previous counseling found that length of therapy was associated with more improvement. Similarly, dose-response studies have suggested that as the number of sessions increases, a greater proportion of clients improve (cf. Meyer et al., 1998). Other reviews, however, find no differences or advantages for brief therapy (Barber, 1994; Steenbarger, 1994).

Problems with contemporary outcome assessment

One explanation for the field's inability to answer complicated questions such as the effects of treatment length is that we continue to use relatively primitive methods to assess outcome. Historically, psychological and educational tests have been created to measure *traits,* stable personal characteristics thought to be largely immune from the effects of situations or development (Meier, 1994). The prototypic trait is intelligence or cognitive ability, a characteristic many psychologists believe is strongly influenced by heredity and relatively stable over the life span. Not surprisingly, the history of educational and psychological testing is largely an account of measures designed to measure intelligence or related constructs such as academic achievement, ability, and aptitude. In contrast, the measurement of outcome is often concerned with measuring *states,* such as anxiety or depression, amenable to change through counseling and psychotherapy (cf. Strupp, Horowitz, & Lambert, 1997).

Current outcome measures

Unfortunately, many of the tests now being employed to measure outcome appear to have been created with the traditional methodologies used to construct tests measuring traits. One of the newest outcome scales, for example, is the Outcome Questionnaire-45 or OQ-45 (Lambert & Huefner, 1996). A 45-item inventory of client-reported distress and symptoms, the OQ-45 produces a total score and scores on three subscales: Symptom Distress, Interpersonal Relations, and Social Role Performance.

One piece of evidence used to support the use of OQ-45 is that it has adequate test-retest reliability (Burlingame, Lambert, Reisinger, Neff, & Mosier, 1995); that is, scores on the scale tend to remain stable over time. Tests that measure therapeutic effects, however, should show change in the presence of an intervention but stability when no intervention is present (Meier, 1997, 1998). While the OQ-45 shows change in response to treatment, a study with college students also indicated that students show improvement on OQ items even when they are not in counseling (Lambert & Huefner, 1996). Similarly, an attempt to confirm the three factors proposed in the original scale was not successful (Mueller, Lambert, & Burlingame, 1998); all three scales were highly intercorrelated. One guess at this early stage of research is that many OQ items are measuring relatively stable personality traits (e.g., neuroticism) instead of the type of states likely to be affected by counseling of a more short-term nature.

More substantial problems are apparent with the Global Assessment of Functioning (GAF; American Psychiatric Association, 1994) scale, perhaps the most widely used outcome measure. The GAF is a one-item 100-point rating scale with which clinicians can summarize a client's overall functioning and symptomatology over daily, weekly, or monthly periods. For outcome assessment, GAF ratings are typically completed at intake and termination. Despite its widespread use, little psychometric data are available for its current form (Basco, Krebaum, and Rush, 1997). Spitzer, Gibbon, Williams, and Endicott (1996), however, noted that researchers have reported modest test-retest reliability values in the .60 to .80 range.

The basic issue with the GAF is its transparency: the rater can easily manipulate the rating, making the client appear as distressed or functional as necessary (cf. Speer & Newman, 1996). Thus, the GAF allows the clinician to justify treatment with an insurer but at a cost of instrument validity. The scatterplot on page 59 displays, over a one-year period at a community mental health center, the number of therapy sessions plotted against GAF intake scores. Theoretically, lower GAF scores, indicating greater severity and dysfunction, should be associated with greater number of visits. The plot shows a triangular shape, however, with the fewest number of visits associated with both the lowest and highest GAF scores. In addition, the clustering of scores in the 40 to 50 range suggests that clinicians have learned what GAF scores they need to obtain and maintain services from insurers.

Counselors seeking to learn about additional measures can consult Clement (1999) and Ogles, Lambert, and Masters (1996).

Satisfaction measures

Another type of measure popular with insurance companies, patient satisfaction, possesses its own set of problems. Satisfaction measures are also very transparent, typically asking clients to rate their happiness with the health care services provided. In our experience with such surveys, providers commonly receive high ratings from clients (cf. Beisecker, 1996; Di Palo, 1998; Lewis, 1994; Sitzia & Wood, 1997; Stallard, 1996). We speculate, only partially facetiously, that one would need to physically harm most mental health clients or medical patients before they would rate the provided service as unsatisfactory (but see Gaston & Sabourin, 1992, and LeBow, 1983, for more sophisticated perspectives). Consequently, we experience considerable skepticism when managed care companies proudly advertise satisfaction ratings in the 50 to 75 percent range. We suspect that any service receiving good or excellent ratings totaling less than 75 percent of the polled clients suffers from some significant problems.

Missing data

An even more basic problem can bedevil the task of collecting outcome assessments: missing data. Outcome data may be missing for a variety of reasons, including client dropout and failure to complete outcome assessments at termination. Speer and Newman (1996) examined outcome evaluation studies conducted in community mental health service settings and found 10 studies whose response rates ranged from 19 percent to 74 percent. Other reviews of outcome studies report similar results: Roback and Smith's (1987) study of eight outpatient psychotherapy groups found a 13 percent to 63 percent attrition range, while Stark (1992) reported even higher dropout rates (from 45 percent to 96 percent) in studies of alcohol and drug treatment. Attrition rates in outpatient counseling with children have been estimated between 40 percent and 60 percent (Kazdin, 1996; Wierzbicki & Pekarik, 1993).

When attrition and missing data are so substantial, the major issue centers on whether the missing data are random or a result of a systematic factor. A considerable body of evidence, for example, indicates that clients who participate in follow-up assessments are generally more functional and

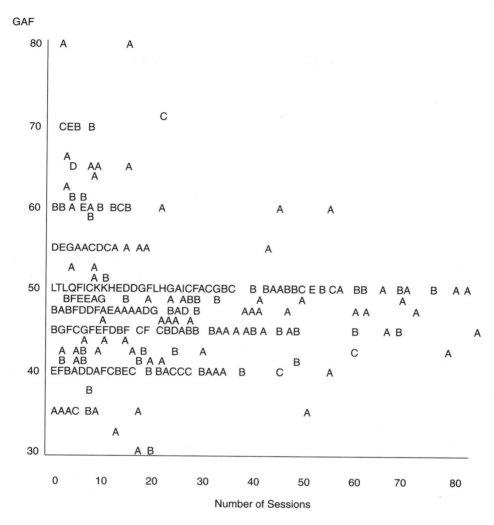

Number of Sessions

Note. Relationship between GAF scores at intake and total number of counseling sessions over a one-year period at a community mental health center. *A* represents one GAF rating, *B* represents two ratings, and so forth. Lower GAF scores, indicating greater severity and dysfunction, should be associated with greater number of visits, but they are not.

have more resources than clients who cannot or do not provide follow-up data (e.g., Epstein, McCrady, Miller, & Steinberg, 1994; Hayslip, Hoffman, & Weatherly, 1990–1991; Norton, Breitner, Welsh, & Wyse, 1994; Speer & Zold, 1971). Similar results have been found in medical studies (Herndon, Fleishman, Kosty, & Green, 1997). Thus, conclusions based on outcome data completed by only a portion of the individuals who received services may be misleading.

Implications for managed care

These measurement and data collection problems bear upon quality issues in managed care. For example, some observers and executives of managed care companies believe that the lack of quality now evident in what they consider the initial phase of the industrialization of health care will soon be replaced by a higher level of service. To the contrary, we predict that an emphasis on higher quality, at least in mental health, will not happen soon for three reasons. First, as described, current outcome measures do not have the necessary precision to give feedback about what works and what does not beyond a broad result; consequently, little valid information currently exists about how to reliably improve counseling and psychotherapy. Second, despite the fact that managed care companies are improving their information-gathering capacities (Cummings, 1996), we strongly suspect that much outcome information so generated will be considered proprietary by those companies and not widely shared with the counseling or research community.

Third, most managed care companies have given no indication that they will be motivated by factors other than profit. Cummings and Sayama (1995) similarly believe that despite a need to demonstrate "efficiency, effectiveness, and quality . . . at the present time, there seems to be an inability on the part of managed care companies to do this convincingly" (p. 40). Based on past behavior, we believe that outcomes such as quality of care will remain distant priorities for managed care companies without the intervention of forces outside the marketplace. Instead, most managed care companies will use outcome assessment as yet another device for denying services and delaying payment for services already rendered.

The press to measure outcome

Despite difficulties with current measures and missing data, funding sources such as managed care companies are increasingly requiring agencies and counselors to conduct outcome assessments to document treatment effectiveness. As Sauber (1997b, pp. 14–15) wrote about the ascendance of managed care:

> The most radical change for therapists will be the need to justify what they do with an unprecedented precision and specificity. Therapists, according to Sykes-Wylie (1994), are held to almost no objectively measurable external standards for deciding what is wrong with the client, what to do about it, how long it should take to do it, when it can be considered done, and how anybody knows if it is done.

Part of the problem is that historically, many laypersons and even some counselors and researchers have believed that the effects of counseling and psychotherapy were essentially too subjective to measure or quantify. The important corollary to this belief, however, is that if mental health services are too subjective to quantify, they may also be too subjective to pay for (Brown, 1991). Clearly the profession needs better methods of measuring outcome, both to justify its worth to outside payors and to advance as a science.

Potential solutions

If current outcome measures are problematic, what are other options? The possibilities include:

- examining decreases in the use of medical services after counseling,
- using intervention-sensitive item selection guidelines to develop new outcome measures,
- increasing the use of idiographic assessment, and
- developing basic quality standards for outcome assessment.

Medical cost offset

Cummings (1996) wrote that "in our society persons in emotional distress very often have somatic symptoms, and reduction in somatization is a reliable measure of diminution of emotional distress in that group of people" (p. 222). Medical offset effects refers to situations in which persons who receive psychotherapy subsequently require fewer medical and surgical services. Given the history of medical cost offset from psychotherapy, Cummings (1996) believes that the degree of reduction in medical utilization can function as an objective measure of outcome not subject to the transparency effects of most self-report measures.

Sauber (1997b), however, warned that everyone from politicians to insurance companies needs to be educated about how mental health contributes to physical health. Thus, the validity of outcome measures that focused on medical use and physical symptoms may not be believable to important parties.

Change-sensitive tests

It should be possible to create tests that more sensitively measure the states influenced by counseling and psychotherapy. Drawing on the concepts described by criterion-referenced and longitudinal test developers (Collins, 1991; Gronlund, 1988; Tryon, 1991), Meier (1997, 1998) developed a set of guidelines for developing such tests. Meier (1998) then conducted a comparison of traditional and change-sensitive versions of an alcohol attitudes scale completed by college students who received one of two experimental conditions (i.e., an alcohol education group or a control group). The intervention-sensitive items did detect pre-post change; these items also possessed lower test-retest reliability in intervention participants while demonstrating stability when completed by controls. In contrast, items evaluated with traditional criteria demonstrated greater internal consistency and variability, characteristics that enhance measurement of stable individual differences. Other studies have also found a difference between change-sensitive items and traditional tests (e.g., Kopta, Howard, Lowry, & Beutler, 1994). In a study of a symptom checklist completed at intake and termination by students at a college counseling center, for example, Weinstock (1999) found similar differences between intervention-sensitive and traditionally selected test items.

So paying attention to the eventual purpose of testing during the test construction phase may result in measures more sensitive to the effects of counseling and psychotherapy. Because of the need for large sample sizes during item selection, such tests would likely be most effective for investigating the outcomes of *groups* of counselors (e.g., at agencies and clinics). These tests should also be useful for investigating more specific questions such as how outcome is influenced when counseling is completed by persons of different age, gender, and race.

Idiographic measures

The third possibility for improving outcome assessment is *idiographic* assessment. An idiographic perspective attempts to understand the uniqueness of the individual client, family, or group and thereby enhance the clinician's understanding and ability to predict future behavior (Meier, 1994). In idiographic assessment the focus of attention are elements relatively specific to the particular individual. A depressed individual, for example, may show symptoms common to others (e.g., sleep disturbance) as well as relatively unique to her- or himself (e.g., a client who claims not to be depressed but reports that he wants to die). Similarly, three clients might predominantly express anxiety as the amount of hair-pulling, sweating, and self-reported tension, respectively.

In contrast, both the OQ-45 and the GAF are nomothetic measures; their items and ratings presumably apply to all individuals in the same way. However, because no individual is likely to display all or just the right combination (i.e., a prototype) of the indicators of a construct, idiographic measures should better indicate change than nomothetic devices. In other words, unless a nomothetic measure has sampled the universe of a construct's indicators—for example, a depression measure that includes items assessing all possible ways an individual could experience or express depression—it may not function with a specific individual as well as an idiographic measure.

In idiographic assessment the assessor/counselor observes how the client manifests constructs important to therapeutic process and outcome. These indicators are likely to become more apparent as the counseling relationship progresses and the client engages in self-exploration and greater sharing of therapeutic material with the counselor. Determining what is important in the rich description of self and world offered by the client is part of the task of case conceptualization. The counselor conceptualizes the client and attempts to find the best indicators of constructs important to this particular person. *Best* in this context includes the most accessible and efficient methods: the counselor may draw upon such diverse sources as the client's self-report, counselor ratings of in-session or other behaviors, or observations by others (e.g., parent or teacher observations of children, staff ratings of inpatient behaviors). Analysis of the resulting data can inform the counselor about the client's progress as well as the validity of the case conceptualization (Meier, 1999).

More specific examples of case conceptualizations and idiographic assessments can be found in *Bridging Case Conceptualization, Assessment, and Intervention* at *www.acsu.buffalo.edu/~stmeier.*

Quality standards for data collection and outcome assessment

In the short term, funding agencies will continue to demand outcome information from individual counselors and the agencies where they work. We think it is important to begin a discussion about what is a reasonable amount and type of information to provide, that is, basic quality standards for data collection and outcome assessment. For example, we suggest that the *degree of missing data* and the *quality of the collected data* be considered additional measures of outcome (Meier & Letsch, in press):

1. Agencies and health care providers might assess their ability to collect post-intake data. While it is often relatively simple to collect data from clients and therapists at intake, the task typically becomes more complex beyond the first session. For example, clients may attend counseling for a few sessions and improve, but then drop out without providing an opportunity to gather a second outcome assessment. Clients may fully complete counseling, but because of a lack of interest on their part or their counselors', fail to complete a second assessment.

   As noted, data collection rates have significant implications for analyses of outcome assessment data. First, low missing data rates strengthen the generalizability of outcome data by suggesting that treatment works across more than simply the healthiest subgroup of clients. Clinicians and agencies with substantial missing data rates should be cautious when reporting positive treatment effects: the widely observed link between client severity and attrition indicates that if analyses were to contain the entire sample of clients who began treatment, findings of client improvement would likely be tempered. In settings with moderate to low data collection rates, it is more valid to conclude that treatment services are effective for the healthier subset who begin and complete treatment than to state that treatment services in general are effective.

   Low data collection rates, even at sites with substantial numbers of clients, may mean that interpretation of the statistical significance of analyses of pre-post change could be hindered by the resulting small sample size. Clinicians should also consider the use of missing data rates from empirical studies (e.g., Meier & Letsch, in press) as baselines for comparison. Improvements in relation to these baselines, as well as improvements over time within the particular field setting, may be selling points to third-party payors. Although no consensus is present regarding minimum levels, Speer and Newman (1996) have recommended a 90 percent data completion rate to strengthen conclusions and suggested that rates below 70 percent should place findings in question.

2. Agencies and individual counselors should consider gathering evidence concerning the quality of their outcome data. Several strategies are available:

   - Calculate basic reliability estimates for outcome assessments completed by their clients (cf. Meier, 1999). Coefficient *alphas* provide an estimate of internal consistency for multiple-item outcome scales; *alphas* below a .70 to .80 range are questionable (cf. Meier & Davis, 1990).

- Gather basic validity evidence by correlating two or more outcome assessments with each other.
- Collect outcome data from multiple sources; missing data rates may vary considerably by source (Meier & Letsch, in press). Convergent outcome results from multiple sources strengthen claims of treatment effectiveness, particularly if one or more of the sources has even the appearance of motivation to overstate treatment effects.

Given this background, Meier and Letsch (in press) proposed the following guideline regarding the level of necessary and sufficient data collection for outcome assessment:

Groups of counselors whose assessments are based on *substantial data collection rates* and include *evidence of data quality* have a sound basis to reject demands for additional record-keeping from third parties.

At the present time, no empirical claim can be made that (a) the collection of large amounts or types of data at intake or subsequent follow-up leads to improved treatment outcome (cf. Hayes, Nelson, & Jarrett, 1987), or (b) any particular outcome scale or set of scales is psychometrically superior to others. Demands for additional record-keeping and information beyond this general standard can only be viewed as disincentives for utilization of services.

Summary

Research relevant to managed care is in an initial stage. For example, much basic research remains to be done on the effects of managed care policies. For example, do gender, age, or racial differences exist in the type or amount of mental health coverage provided to individuals? Similarly, the mental health professions would benefit from improved methods of measuring therapeutic progress and outcome. Such measures could benefit counselors and clients by providing information about when and how to adjust the provided intervention. Counselors have been criticized for providing no external data to substantiate their clinical judgments. At the same time, insurers have no strong basis for making treatment decisions with individual clients (e.g., approving or denying care, or types of treatment) on the basis of current tests. Better measures of outcome could usefully serve as an aid to clinical judgment *and* quality indicators of interest to managed care companies.

Can Managed Care Be Improved?

Managed care companies often seem determined to avoid changing the fundamental ways they do business. One managed care executive, for example, claimed that "the perceived failings of managed care have been loudly and widely expressed and based largely on anecdotal evidence" (Major, 1999, p. 1). As part of this chapter will make clear, however, better research is beginning to appear concerning the effects of managed care, and it supports much of the "anecdotal evidence" that managed care executives would like to dismiss.

This chapter is clearly the most opinionated of the book, but we have written it because we believe the mental health professions must unite and work with other professions that share our people-oriented values. We present evidence to support our positions and invite the reader to consider these issues in depth.

Is basic health care a right?

"No" seems to be the reply of many in the corporate world and their legislative procurers, who neither want to pay more for employer-provided health care nor support efforts for government-sponsored programs. "Yes" is the reply of nearly everyone else, including persons sympathetic to managed care. For example, Cummings and Sayama (1995, p. 30) wrote that "Our health-care system will eventually have to be universal in its delivery. . . . To put it simply, everyone will have shoes, but there will be no Gucci loafers." The issue of fairness in the health care system needs to be put on the agenda (Daniels et al., 1996).

Specialists in health economics, Giles (1993) reported, have pointed to an emphasis on ethics and human rights—characteristic of Western cultures especially—as the "culprit" in the health care crisis. Health care in the United States is considered, in principle at least, to be a right available to all. Giles (1993) concluded that "all are of the opinion that providers, left unregulated in a fee-for-service environment, will take advantage of this fiscal system until health care becomes unobtainable except for the privileged" (p. 22). Six years after this was published it is becoming apparent that at least in the area of mental health services, the opposite is true: Managed care companies increasingly constrict services to cut costs, and many of the clients remaining in therapy in settings such as community agencies and private practice are paying out-of-pocket. The poor and uninsured have been lost in this debate: At present over 40 million Americans lack basic health insurance (Finkelstein, 1997).

Another way of asking this question is: Are the enormous profits being made by many corporations more important than providing basic health, education, and social services? In addition to cutting costs, DeLeon et al. (1994) noted that in recent years HMOs have been used "as a means of . . . providing investment opportunities" (p. 33). Managed care companies have been profiting enormously over the past decade (Kuttner, 1999). For example, PacifiCare grew from a $168,911 company in 1986 to a $10 billion giant by 1997 (Glasser, 1998). The Associated Press reported that United Healthcare Corporation in 1994 paid each member of its Board of Directors $109,000 per meeting. The total per member for the year was $981,500. Similarly, the Albany (NY) *Times Union* (May 7, 1995) reported huge increases in 1994 to salaries paid to executives of HMOs; one executive earned $241,140 in 1994, up 36 percent from the previous year. Given this kind of money, it is no surprise that HMOs object to rules requiring them to publish executive salaries or information about their medical loss ratios.

Given this kind of money, we find some of the current debates in the U.S. Congress about health care reform ridiculous. For example, in 1999 Congress was arguing about the merits of health care legislation proposed by Democratic representatives that would cover all Americans, provide the right to sue health plans, and ensure easier access to care (Meckler, 1999). The major controversy centered on whether the reform would increase health insurance premiums by 4.8 percent (the Democrats' estimate) or 6.1 percent (the Republicans' estimate)—a difference of 1.3 percent.

Values

Perhaps the most basic reason that the realms of counseling and managed care appear worlds apart is their respective set of work values. While "the managed-care process is motivated predominantly by economics" (Sauber, 1997b, p. 8), most health care professionals believe that the "pursuit of corporate profit and personal fortune have no place in caregiving" (Ad Hoc Committee to Defend Health Care, 1997, p. 1733). Similarly, Miller (1998) concluded that "perhaps it will eventually appear blindingly obvious that acceding to the short-term profit taking and unbridled competition of managed care and merger mania is a mistake" (p. 473).

In 1980, the average CEO in *Business Week*'s annual survey made 42 times as much as a factory worker. By 1997, the average CEO was making 326 times as much. The average CEO of a major corporation made $7.8 million, 326 times the $24,000 earned by the average factory worker (Jackson, 1999). A Families USA study of MCO executive compensation found that in 1996, the 25 highest paid HMO executives had an average compensation over $6.2 million (see *www.hmopage.org*). In 1985 nearly two-thirds of all businesses with one hundred or more employees paid the full cost of health care coverage. Despite the fact that 80 percent of Americans believe that employers should be required to offer health insurance (Corcoran & Vandiver, 1996), fewer than one-third still do. In contrast, a recent *New Yorker* article (Auletta, 1999) provides an idea about the kind of health care some CEOs expect. During a river rafting trip at a summer camp for CEOs and their families in Sun Valley, Idaho, ambulances followed the group *in case* someone got hurt.

At a more psychological level, many counselors are disturbed that managed care decision-makers approach their work as if it were a competitive sport. Health care is approached as a win/lose proposition (cf. Kessler, 1998) and power is wielded to be certain managed care *wins.* In the area of mental health services, managed care companies historically have avoided negotiations and simply employed their economic power to impose changes. As Giles (1993) put it, managed care "represents the attempt by corporations to wrest much of the control of the payment and provision of treatment services from those who have traditionally provided it" (p. 1). More bluntly, Sauber (1997b, p. 14) cites Shulman as describing the difference between a terrorist and a managed care company: "You can negotiate with a terrorist."

Will managed care evolve?

Some observers argue that managed care companies are already beginning to compete with each other based on quality and service as well as cost (e.g., Newman & Reed, 1996). However, if companies continue to consolidate at the present rate, there may be little competition left to spur movement beyond the current cost overemphasis. Only four corporations in the late 1980s owned 59 percent of all private for-profit hospitals (Bickman & Dokecki, 1989; Browskowski, 1994). Similarly, some argue that capitation will motivate companies to emphasize prevention and health promotion (e.g., Newman & Reed, 1996). This assumes, however, that executives in managed care companies will do the hard work of establishing effective prevention programs and not simply slash services further to boost the bottom lines of their companies.

Who will evaluate managed care?

Research on the effects of managed care is in its infancy, prompting the observation that "it seems ironic that the external parties demanding accountability have little evidence of their own effectiveness" (Corcoran & Vandiver, 1996, p. 35). Yet the studies that have been done indicate that managed care has not improved health care (Jost, 1998).

A recent study published in the *Journal of the American Medical Association* reported that for-profit HMOs provided worse care than non-profit HMOs on all 14 quality-of-care dimensions that were studied (Himmelstein, Woolhandler, Hellander, & Wolfe, 1999; Galewitz, 1999a). Among the quality-of-care dimensions were infant immunization, mammography, pap smear, early prenatal care, and beta-blockers for heart patients. The authors report the largest differences were present for care following hospitalization for heart attack (i.e., use of beta-blockers) and diabetes.

The study employed data from the National Committee for Quality Assurance (NCQA), a group composed of health-plan representatives and employers that accredits managed care companies, and included the Health Plan Employer Data and Information Set (HEDIS), a set of standard measures designed to compare health plans. The data reflect performance in 329 HMO plans (248 for-profit and 81 nonprofit) in 45 states in 1996; this represents just over half of all HMO enrollment in the United States.

Himmelstein et al. (1999) found that nonprofits spend 86.9 percent of their revenues on medical and hospital services compared to 80.6 percent of for-profits. This means that spending on profit and administrative overhead was nearly 50 percent higher in for-profit plans compared to nonprofits (19.4 percent versus 13.1 percent). Despite these differences, the authors noted that many more people have been enrolling over the past 15 years in for-profit plans than nonprofit. The cost per HMO member per month averaged $128 in for-profit and $127.50 in nonprofit plans. Himmelstein et al. (1999) also criticized the HEDIS quality indicators. None of the indicators measure outcome, instead focusing on inexpensive preventive services; HEDIS indicators also fail to address quality issues for the seriously and chronically ill.

From a methodological perspective, this study is remarkable on two fronts. First, all 14 quality-of-life indicators demonstrate an advantage for nonprofit HMOs. No ambiguity exists here, unlike many research findings, and the consistency of these results indicates that the nonprofit advantage is likely to generalize to other measures. The differences are also likely to grow larger when the sample studied includes more seriously and chronically ill individuals. Second, these data were provided from the managed care association's database. If any bias were present, we would expect the results to minimize the managed care companies' position that for-profit and nonprofit companies provide care of equal quality. These data likely underestimate the quality of care provided by nonprofit companies compared to for-profit insurers.

A recent *Consumer Reports* survey of 19,000 readers confirmed the common belief that persons with health problems are more likely to have trouble with their HMO than healthy persons in that HMO (Lieberman, 1999). *Consumer Reports* found that in the lowest-ranked health plans, persons with serious health problems were about three times as likely as healthy persons to report trouble obtaining care from their HMO. Even in highly ranked plans, however, persons with health problems were twice as likely to report such difficulty.

Another recent study indicated that both doctors and patients are very frustrated in their attempts to obtain needed care from HMOs. CBS News reported on a Kaiser Family Foundation survey of 1,053 doctors and 768 nurses during February and June 1999. Eighty-seven percent of the doctors reported that patients had been denied some type of service over the previous two years. Of particular interest is that 38 percent of the doctors reported having difficulty obtaining a mental health or substance abuse referral for their patients. Doctors indicated that these denials often led to a serious decline in health. Another finding of interest is that about 30 percent of doctors and nurses reported exaggerating patient symptoms to receive needed treatment.

Many states have begun to publish report cards comparing different managed care companies. These evaluations, however, are so rudimentary in nature that they provide little basis for consumers to make choices or for government agencies to provide regulation (cf. Leff & Woocher, 1997; Lieberman, 1999). We predict that while quality-of-care indicators will most interest providers and patients, the major aspect of performance that will interest MCOs is what they will define as overutilization of services (cf. Magellan Behavioral Health, 1999, a description provided by a MCO of NCQA and HEDIS). In addition, any evaluation procedures should be explicitly public (Daniels et al., 1996).

Specific suggestions

Experts continue to offer a variety of broad proposals for improving health care, such as the establishment of democratic procedures for allocating health care resources, fair grievance procedures, and increased respect for confidentiality and privacy (Daniels et al., 1996). We now consider specific actions that have the potential to improve the health care system and managed care. Seven pragmatic directions are summarized that could make a significant impact.

Continue the transition from inpatient to outpatient services

This is probably the single most important step to take to reduce costs in mental health services (cf. Richardson & Austad, 1994). Given that (a) much more money is spent on inpatient care than outpatient and that (b) little or no evidence supports the general efficacy of inpatient treatment over out-patient treatment, it makes sense that managed care companies should seek providers and programs who minimize the need for inpatient services and rehospitalization (Mechanic, 1997).

Mechanic (1997) suggested that the major source of financial savings for managed care companies has indeed been to reduce inpatient admissions and longer length of stays. However, managed care companies have also reduced outpatient services.

Simplify the managed care and medical bureaucracy

In the mental health arena, Sauber (1997) recommended that we (a) end managed care's micromanagement of individual cases and (b) set rational guidelines for care. This implies a renewed emphasis on research to provide a foundation for treatment decisions. Managed care, for example, should provide data to answer such questions as, "Does utilization review add to the quality of services?" Regarding treatment decisions, empirically-validated treatments (EVTs) and accompanying treatment manuals are specific counseling approaches that have been shown to produce effective outcomes for particular client problems (Pikoff, 1996; Meier & Davis, 2000). It might make sense, for example, to review only those therapists or cases that routinely exceed the number of sessions recommended for particular problems and their EVTs.

Other managed care processes can be simplified (Sauber, 1997b). The complex process of appealing most companies' treatment decisions now discourages such appeals, particularly for persons with severe problems. Consider rewarding therapists for patient satisfaction and outcome as well as cost, and return cost savings to the patients and employers who pay the bills.

Invest in research

Economics, not science, drives contemporary managed care. Yet the results of better research into counseling processes and outcomes offer hope for improving practice and reducing cost. Among the wide range of questions needing attention are:

- As noted in Chapter 4, how can we construct better measures of outcome?
- Do particular counseling approaches work better with persons who have specific problems such as depression or schizophrenia? If so,

how do factors such as client age, gender, and ethnicity influence the results?

- What type of health care organizations best balance concerns about quality *and* cost (cf. Corcoran & Vandiver, 1996)? Similarly, what types of private-public organizations work best?

- What are the effects of using "medical necessity" as the criteria for providing services to persons with mental health issues? Would "psychosocial necessity" be more appropriate (cf. Vandivort-Warren, 1998)?

- If underutilization is occurring, how would its effects be apparent (Daniels, Light, & Caplan, 1996)?

- Are measures of client satisfaction valid? That is, what factors influence scores on satisfaction measures?

Private and public agencies such as the Agency for Health Care Policy Research need support to conduct and sponsor research that addresses such questions.

Remove control of health insurance from employers

Shore (1996) proposed that employers no longer pay health insurance premiums, but that employees use that money to purchase their own health care plans. She suggests that government pay the balance of fees for unemployed persons or those with limited incomes. Shore also argues for use of Medical Savings Accounts (MSAs) whose funds are employed for medical expenses. With MSAs individuals make tax-free deposits and withdraw money without penalty to pay medical expenses or health insurance premiums. MSA money could be used to pay for routine, smaller medical bills while catastrophic coverage would be covered by more traditional health insurance. MSAs have been projected to lower administrative health care costs and thus save the U.S. health care system almost $600 billion over five years (see *www.hmopage.org/msawhat.html*). MSAs also increase choice in the medical marketplace by giving health care money to patients.

Consider staffing ratios

Many problems with managed care companies stem from their push to perform tasks with a minimum complement of employees. From insufficient billing staff to cutbacks of nurses in hospitals, managed care attempts to maximize profits by minimizing personnel. States such as California have been considering legislation to set regulations on minimum nurse-patient ratios. While it may be impractical to regulate the number of claims clerks, considerable research and discussion is needed to set standards about the number and type of employees and professionals needed within managed care companies and in health care settings to insure quality services. Accreditation bodies appear to have set the bar too low for managed care companies.

In a similar vein, some managed care advocates tout the increasing use of computer technology as improving the efficiency of billing services. Fox (1997) noted that such technology typically lowers administrative costs and provides a vehicle for gathering information about providers and the costs associated with different diagnoses. While such systems should also increase the efficiency of processing and paying claims, the examples provided earlier in this book indicate that in mental health they often do not. Like everyone else, managed care companies should pay their bills on time.

Consider traditional labor strategies

Some of the approaches employed historically by labor unions may be useful for dealing with managed care. For example, the New York State Psychological Association recently joined a large teacher's union in an effort to gain the union's expertise and strength in (a) potential bargaining with managed care companies and (b) lobbying government officials (Dean & Feder, 1999).

Although a high-stakes move in today's political climate, groups of mental health professionals employed by a managed care company may also consider a strike. In 1998, 54 mental health professionals employed by Kaiser Permanente of Colorado held a one-day strike to protest the heavy caseloads they were experiencing (McGuire, 1998). The therapists were protesting the company's decision to add 10 additional clients per week in addition to their regular caseload. The additional caseload meant delays for clients in beginning therapy and difficulty for clients seeking to see their therapists on a regular schedule.

Offer or attend classes on managed care

Given managed care's impact on the profession, counselor educators should consider how best to integrate information about managed care into the curriculum (Davidson, 1998). Many mental health programs and educators appear to have underestimated managed care's impact and are now behind in their efforts to keep students current about managed care (cf. Davis, 1998). While a separate course may be optimal for educating students (Brooks & Riley, 1998), managed care content can easily fit into ethical, legal, health policy, practicum, and counseling courses. Courses with managed care content (e.g., including policy, political, and practice components) are likely to be of interest to current students as well as recent graduates.

ⓥ *Be politically active*

The reactions of many counselors to the loss of autonomy and increased workload imposed by managed care range from rage to helplessness. That is, many helping professionals can be characterized as either fighting managed care or adapting to it. Even the reviewers of the first draft of this book evidenced this range of response. One reviewer wrote that:

> Clearly clinicians must learn to work with managed care. Even if it is an evil, it is one with which we must learn to dance.

Interestingly, another reviewer suggested the opposite:

> I wish the authors had indicated, from the beginning, that some clinicians decline to play the MCO game, and that this option also has certain advantages.

Shore (1996) is among those fighting managed care. She argues that managed care deprives individuals of the right to:

- choose their clinicians, pharmacies, and treatment facilities,
- make their own treatment decisions, and
- decide what medical information is recorded and who has the right to access it.

Shore (1996) believes that:

> Consumer freedom and managed care are inimical to each other. Managed care controls costs by controlling the behavior of clinicians and patients. Their cost-containment mechanisms require limits on consumer choice and freedom, and that clinicians not advocate for patients. (p. 24)

Clearly there has been a short-term price to pay for those who have fought managed care. For example, Cummings and Sayama (1995, p. 19) wrote that:

> The American Psychological Association (APA) deluded itself into believing it could be a David confronting Goliath. Persisting in its strenuous opposition, the APA has rendered itself irrelevant and is being cut out of the decision-making process within the industry.

At the level of individual providers, Kongstvedt (1997) advised managed care managers who encounter "noncompliant" (p. 401) physicians to cut them out of the plan:

> If education and personal appeals [to the provider] fail to effect the needed change, you must take action. Failure to take action is the mark of weak and ineffectual management. (p. 401)

In contrast to active resistance, the prevalent stance taken in the professional literature has been to adapt to managed care. For example, Sauber (1997, p. xii) maintained that clinicians "have to stop grieving for what was and move from denial to anger to acceptance to cooperation! Managed care is here to stay." Some counselors also feel like the victims of managed care. Kassan (1996) quoted one therapist who said:

> Managed care is a nightmare. We're no longer doctors, we're providers. . . . It's political, and I'm not a political person. It's very depressing to see this happening and be a victim of it, and to see my clients be victims of it, because they are. (p. 551)

Our suggestion is that counselors not simply adapt *or* fight, but adapt *and* fight. Most counselors, for a number of reasons, cannot escape working with managed care or a managed care philosophy; we hope these professionals can use many of this book's strategies to cope with specific managed care practices. In addition, one of the conclusions we have reached after dealing with and researching managed care is that more counselors must push themselves to become politically active (cf. Haynes & Mickelson, 2000; Welch, 1999). Even if that prospect is not appealing to you, we suggest that at a minimum, you at least join a professional organization and support that group with dues (Buchholz, 1998). From there you can decide whether to become more active with local, regional, and national groups who deal with managed care. For example, many professional organizations and other groups fighting managed care need donations of time and money. Managed care companies and related health care associations have huge amounts of money available to them to influence public opinion and legislators at every level (cf. Daniels et al., 1996). In the summer of 1999, for example, media reports indicated that managed care companies were gearing up a $9 million ad campaign to influence the Congressional debate on health care reform.

Health care professionals are becoming increasingly visible to the public regarding their experiences with managed care. One recent event was "Rescue Health Care Day" held on April 1, 2000. This event included teach-ins, an hour of protest, and a minute of silence designed to educate people about managed care, protest its abuses, and begin discussing alternate systems.

Stay informed

Part of being politically active means keeping abreast of the swiftly changing events related to managed care. Newspapers, television stations, and other media tend to be sporadic in their coverage, often focusing on controversy and reporting in little depth about important issues. Counselors will need to be active in their attention to managed care issues. One of the best examples of what *not* to do was related by a colleague who was a member of a professional organization's committee on managed care. The committee was looking for assistance and approached a private practitioner about his willingness to join the group. His response: "How much will you pay me?"

Professional journals such as the *American Psychologist, Journal of the American Medical Association,* and *Administration and Policy in Mental Health* are important resources for managed care information (see Corcoran & Vandiver, 1996, p. 238, for a more complete list). The Internet has become one of the best methods of staying up-to-date on current events and the topic of managed care is no exception. A number of groups specifically interested in managed care issues maintain websites, including:

www.amso.com— American Medical Specialty Organization, Inc., is a managed care company, and this site primarily provides managed care information to their providers and consumers.

www.tiac.net/biz/drmike/Managed2.html This site contains an interview with Nicholas Cummings, a psychologist with pro-managed care views, speculating on the future outlook for managed care and the helping professions.

www.hmopage.com This Physicians Who Care site includes information as well as "Managed Care Horror Stories" and the "Managed Care Hall of Shame."

www.ahcpr.gov A site describing the work of the Agency for Healthcare Research and Quality, which examines health care policy and effects of managed care.

www.policy.com/vcongress/pbor/index.html Contains information about the Patient Bill of Rights.

babydoc.home.pipeline.com/mcout.htm A site with managed care web links, with an emphasis on the doctor-patient relationship.

www.nationalcpr.org A site sponsored by the Coalition for Patient Rights that discusses health care privacy issues.

www.nationalpartnership.org This National Partnership for Women and Families site includes articles supporting the Patient Bill of Rights and links to a variety of other websites, including the American Women's Medical Association, the Feminist Women's Health Center, and the National Committee for Quality Assurance.

www.nimh.nih.gov The National Institute of Mental Health provides information regarding education, training, and research. A recent U.S.

Surgeon General's report on mental health and problems funding mental health treatment is available here.

www.NoManagedCare.org   The National Coalition of Mental Health Professionals and Consumers provides relevant information.

www.patientadvocacy.org   More information, from the Center for Patient Advocacy.

Many professional organizations maintain websites that often contain information on managed care:

www.aamft.org   American Association of Marriage and Family Therapists

www.apa.org   American Psychological Association

www.counseling.org   American Counseling Association

www.naspweb.org   National Association of School Psychologists

www.naswdc.org   National Association of Social Workers

www.nbcc.org   National Board of Certified Counselors

www.psych.org   American Psychiatric Association

www.psychologicalscience.org   American Psychological Society

We also recommend that you support organizations that promote campaign finance reform (such as Common Cause, *www.commoncause.org*). Managed care has maintained its influence over the legislative and executive branches of government through well-timed (and large) political donations and public relations campaigns.

All of these addresses (which we will update periodically) can be accessed from the second author's homepage:

www.acsu.buffalo.edu/~stmeier/

Summary

We concluded this chapter on improving managed care with sections on *Political activism* and *Stay informed* because we believe, particularly with mental health decisions, that managed care companies rarely change from within. When UnitedHealth decided to drop its utilization review for physicians in the fall of 1999, for example, the insurer did not extend this shift to mental health benefits (Galewitz, 1999b). As one reviewer of this book wrote: "We will always be in an adversarial relationship with MCOs if we advocate for access to all legitimate services."

While the media may focus some attention on problems associated with managed care, the most likely vehicle for change is government at the state and federal levels. A recent U.S. Surgeon General's report (*www.nimh. nih.gov*) found that (a) one in five Americans experience significant mental health problems, (b) difficulty paying for mental health treatment stops millions from seeking help, and (c) even individuals with health insurance find that plans often pay for little treatment. Such problems led, in 1999, to 27,000 bills in state legislatures designed to fix health care problems (Goldberg, 2000). When government has leveled the playing field, other directions and solutions for the provision of mental health services may have a chance of being negotiated and implemented.

Even when federal or state legislators eventually pass laws to lessen managed care's power, mental health professionals will have to remain alert. One lesson that became clear to us as we wrote this book is that it is time to set aside territorial concerns in the health care and helping professions. Mental health professionals share more core values with other health care professionals (such as physicians, nurses, occupational therapists, and dentists) than we do with managed care executives. Counselors, social workers, psychologists, and psychiatrists have strong reasons to bond together in the struggle with managed care. In our discussions with helping professionals—whether they work in an agency, school, hospital, private practice, or elsewhere—we encounter an amazing similarity of problems. At a political level, we believe the mental health professions must unite and work with other professions that share our people-oriented values.

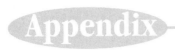

Introduction to Managed Care Terms

Managed care brings with it many new terms and acronyms. Given their origins in the business and financial arenas, many will be unfamiliar to counselors and clinicians.

In this Appendix we describe an essential vocabulary necessary for understanding the basics of managed care. While the Glossary contains a slightly longer list of these and additional terms in alphabetical order, here they are organized by themes. The themes are:

- Organizations
- Who's Insured?
- Providers
- What's Covered?
- Legal and Ethical Issues
- Traditional Insurance
- Assessment and Evaluation
- Cost-Containment
- Legislation and Regulation

Each theme contains a brief explanation and accompanying terms.

Organizations

A dizzying array of acronyms has been created to describe the variety of managed care and related organizations. One of the most basic distinctions that can be made between these organizations is whether they provide insurance (to pay for health care), the health care itself, or a combination of the two.

These organizations often differ by their primary methods of controlling costs. The basic types include:

Health Maintenance Organization (HMO): Any managed care group that provides third-party payment to a provider for services rendered to a voluntarily enrolled prescriber. HMOs may also deliver services directly through their own health care providers.

Managed Care Organizations (MCO): The oversight of medical or mental health care delivery by a third party whose purpose is to limit the care to that which is deemed medically necessary.

Third-party payers: An organization or company responsible for paying providers for services rendered to persons who have contracted with the organization for the management of their health care services. Rather than paying directly for services provided, members pay the organization a fixed amount of money in exchange for guaranteed amounts and types of services.

Individual or Independent Practice Association (IPA): Major HMOs contract with IPAs to provide services to their members. IPAs then contract with practitioners or groups of practitioners who are reimbursed on either a fee-for-service or capitated basis.

Preferred Provider Organization (PPO): A type of managed care system in which the clients are given financial incentive or required to utilize a specific set of providers (i.e., those formally approved by the company) versus another provider of the clients' choice.

National Committee for Quality Assurance (NCQA): A private, nonprofit group predominantly composed of representatives from managed care companies and employers designed to evaluate the quality of managed care plans. NCQA accredits managed care organizations on the basis of a standardized review; they began accrediting MCOs in 1991.

Health Care Finance Agency (HCFA): The federal agency that oversees all health financing policies for Medicare and the Office of Prepaid Health Care. Decisions made by HCFA often result in similar decisions by managed care agencies regarding the standard financial worth of each type of service.

Who's insured?

The cost of health care largely depends upon the characteristics of the individuals receiving it. For example, we would expect older persons to need more care than younger ones. These characteristics can figure into the cost-cutting methods created by managed care. The accompanying procedures and players include:

Cherry picking: Situations where managed care company places exclusions on benefits in their policies so that only the healthiest persons will apply for/accept the policy.

Carve-outs: The separation or carving out of a specific type of health care from the total insurance package. For example, some companies convinced employers that mental health services were so unique that only insurance companies who focused solely on mental health were able to competently administer insurance services in this area. Thus, mental health was carved out from the remaining medical services offered by the insurance company.

Providers

If you think about health care as an industry, all professionals who deliver services can be considered *providers*. To cut costs, managed care companies typically limit the number and type of providers they allow to provide health care. These decisions can have a number of consequences, including ethical ones:

Provider: The health care professional delivering services to members of a managed care company.

Gatekeeper: Usually the primary care provider or HMO representative. A person who first assesses the patient's needs and determines if care from a specialist, a higher costing provider, is necessary. The gatekeeper often provides care of the illness rather than sending the patient to another provider.

Conflict of interest: The division of loyalty between two or more parties that influences the decision-making capacity of the provider. The conflict may bias decisions against one party, particularly when financial advantages occur for choosing one loyalty over the other. The provider, for example, may make money in some instances by not delivering an expensive service to clients.

Provider panel: The managed care company's list of acceptable providers, that is, providers who have contracted to provide services to a managed care company's members. One way to control costs is to establish a small panel of providers and make it expensive or impossible for patients to obtain care from nonpanel providers.

Closed vs. open provider panels: Panels are groups of providers authorized by a managed care company to deliver care; a closed panel consists of a set of providers who exclusively deliver services, such that consumers may not see other providers and independent providers will not receive referrals. Closed panels can be too small to meet the demand of clients, thereby discouraging the use of services.

No-cause panel termination: A managed care company's removal of a provider from its panel without showing justification.

Like-provider provision: State statutes may include this requirement for persons on utilization review panels to be health care providers who are specifically trained and licensed in the health care area for which they review services rendered.

Co-payment: The fee that the patient must pay to the provider for the service/visit separate from any fees the patient pays the HMO or managed care company. The patient's out-of-pocket expense paid directly to the provider is usually either a fixed dollar amount or percentage of the service cost. Co-payment for mental health services is usually much higher than for medical treatment.

What's covered?

Managed care does exactly that: it attempts to control health care costs through the management of treatment-related decisions. Thus, another avenue for cost-cutting centers on the definitions of covered services and approved treatments:

Medical necessity: The threshold or standard determination needed for services to be reimbursed by managed care systems. These services are required for or deemed necessary and appropriate for the diagnosis and treatment of medical conditions.

Acute mental illness: Short-term and time-limited illness. Illness that the insurance company considers resolvable.

Chronic mental illness: Long-term illness that may require ongoing care over an extended period of time. Often not covered by managed care plans.

Mental health benefits: Designated and delineated by the managed care system, those services for which the consumer can/will receive reimbursement.

Short-term therapy: Eight to twelve sessions, often referred to as brief psychotherapy.

Very short-term therapy: Two to four sessions, often the result of HMO's limitations to services.

Continuity of care: The provision of services to a patient such that care is not interrupted or halted for periods of time. For example, managed care rarely pays for sufficient sessions that the client can afford to see a therapist weekly.

Legal and ethical issues

Controlling costs through managing health care can quickly open up legal and ethical problems. Clients and counselors, subsequently, may often find themselves confronted with issues such as:

Gag clauses: Portions of a contract that prevent the therapist from discussing with the client treatment possibilities not covered by the insurance plan.

Hold-harmless provision: Many managed care or health maintenance organizations have providers sign this clause in their contract indicating that the managed care organization will not be held liable for services rendered by the provider.

Yellow-dog contracts: Labor agreements designed for and by employers with the main or sole purpose of meeting the employers' needs. The needs of the employees are ignored.

Wickline v. State of California (1987): Court case which made it the provider's responsibility to push insurance companies for adequate care. In this case, which involved physical rather than mental health care liability in managed care contexts, the court's decision set the principle for imposing liability on the treating physician for not protesting aggressively the third-party payor's limitations to patient care when those limitations impose upon the physician's medical judgment.

Informed consent: Mental health providers obtain consent to provide therapy or perform other related procedures from their patients. Informed consent entails that the patient has adequate mental capacity to provide consent, has obtained sufficient knowledge about the procedure(s), has not experienced any coercion or pressure, either direct or indirect, during the decision-making process, and has documented the decision.

Traditional insurance

With traditional insurance the concern is typically focused on managing the claims process instead of managing health care. Although traditional approaches to providing insurance have been declining, we are aware of companies who have resurrected these methods:

Fee-for-service: A form of financial reimbursement to the provider based on a set rate for each service rendered; the client selected the provider and received treatment without the insurer's prior approval. This was the traditional way of paying for treatment before managed care, and many counselors in private practice still employ this method for individuals who self-pay.

Indemnity insurance: Fee-for-service insurance that allows clients to select providers and obtain treatment without the prior approval of the insurer.

Assessment and evaluation

Improving quality through evaluation and outcome assessment has been one of the promises of managed care. The basic idea is that information about the effects of treatment decisions on outcomes can be used as feedback to improve subsequent decisions. These efforts, however, are only in their infancy:

Quality assurance: The establishment of standards of care and the periodic assessment of the appropriateness of those standards.

Health Plan Employer Data and Information Set (HEDIS): Group of standard measures designed to evaluate health plans.

Outcome assessment: A method designed to gauge the client's level of progress in therapy (i.e., counseling outcome).

Global Assessment of Functioning Scale (GAF): Used for outcome assessment, a scale designed to provide a universal system for clinicians to rank a patient's composite social, occupational, and psychological functioning from a low of zero to a high of 100. Insurers often use GAF to determine whether problem severity is sufficient to merit services. Basic disadvantage of the GAF is its transparency: providers can easily distort the numbers needed to obtain services from health plan.

Medical offset effects: Instance where the provision of mental health services can lead to reduced use of other medical services. For example, treating clients' depression may lead to fewer visits to the emergency room and to general practitioners. Proposed as an objective measure of outcome.

Idiographic assessment: Measurements where the focus of attention are elements relatively specific to a particular individual. A depressed person, for example, may exhibit that depression in a unique way. Proposed as a potentially more precise measure of outcome.

Empirically validated treatments (EVTs): Specific counseling approaches that have been shown through research to produce effective outcomes for particular client problems.

*"Per thousand" statistic: Often referred to during evaluations of days of inpatient use. Equals **Number** of incidents (e.g., admits, visits) occurring in one month divided by total **Enrollment** times 1,000, or 12,000 for annualized statistics; for example, **N/E** × 12,000. This allows comparison of utilized services across time periods.*

Cost-containment

The most direct methods employed by managed care companies to control costs include:

Capitation: A form of reimbursement intended to contain health care costs by limiting payment to a fixed amount per person in the population. This fixed amount is assigned to the provider regardless of the actual rate of use of services. This shifts financial risk from the payer (e.g., insurer or employer) to the provider as well as providing an incentive for the provider to provide the least amount of services.

Utilization review: The review of clinical information to determine the medical necessity and appropriateness of services and ensure their cost-effective provision.

Case managers: Person who has primary responsibility in planning, securing, monitoring, and evaluating service provision.

Medical loss ratios: How much money a managed care company spends on health care compared to their profits.

Legislation and regulation

Although we suggest that state and federal government may be the only institution with the power to regulate managed care, historically government has been as interested as business in restricting health care costs through managed care. Among their relevant actions:

The Employee Retirement Income Securities Act (ERISA, 1974): Federal legislation designed to protect workers' retirement plans. However, one effect of ERISA is the prevention of any (a) legal action being brought against and (b) government regulations being imposed upon a company that contracts to provide benefits in the workplace.

Fully insured plans: These are plans where an employer pays for an insurance policy to cover employees' health care. ERISA applies to these plans; contrast with self-insured plans, when an employer pays directly for employees' health care.

HMO Act of 1973: Federal legislation that provided $325 million over a five-year period to encourage the startup of new HMOs and the slowing of health care costs. The 1973 HMO act also allowed profit-oriented corporations to become involved in HMOs.

Diagnosis Related Groups (DRGs): DRGs describe categories of illnesses that might be treated within a certain time frame. DRGs meant that Medicare and Medicaid reimbursement would be based on the diagnosis of the patient instead of the previous formula of cost plus profit.

If you understand these terms, you now possess the basic vocabulary necessary to understand much of the literature and experiences concerning counseling with managed care. That will be particularly useful when reading the chapters in this text.

Glossary

Here we present a relatively brief glossary of the most important and frequently employed terms. Sources include Austad (1996), Giles (1993), Lowman and Resnick (1994), Rochefort (1997), Pedulla and Rocke (1999), and Sauber (1997a).

Acute mental illness: Short-term and time-limited illness. Illness that the insurance company considers resolvable.

Capitation: A form of reimbursement intended to contain health care costs by limiting payment to a fixed amount per person in the population. This fixed amount is assigned to the provider regardless of the actual rate of use of services. This shifts financial risk from the payer to the provider as well as providing an incentive for the provider to provide the least amount of services.

Carve-outs: The separation or carving out of a specific type of health care from the total insurance package. For example, some companies convinced employers that mental health services were so unique that only insurance companies who focused solely on mental health were able to competently administer insurance services in this area. Thus, mental health was carved out from the remaining medical services offered by the insurance company.

Case managers: Person who has primary responsibility in planning, securing, monitoring, and evaluating service provision.

Cherry picking: Situations where managed care company places exclusions on benefits in their policies so that only the healthiest persons will apply for/accept the policy.

Chronic mental illness: Long-term illness that may require ongoing care over an extended period of time.

Closed vs. open provider panels: Panels are groups of providers authorized by a managed care company to deliver care; a closed panel consists of a set of providers who exclusively deliver services, such that consumers may not see other providers and independent providers will not receive referrals. Closed panels can be too small to meet the demand of clients, thereby discouraging the use of services.

Conflict of interest: The division of loyalty between two or more parties that influences the decision-making capacity of the provider and may bias decisions against one party, particularly when financial advantages occur for choosing one loyalty over the other.

Continuity of care: The provision of services to a patient such that care is not interrupted or halted for periods of time.

Co-payment: The fee that the patient must pay to the provider for the service/visit separate from any fees the patient pays the HMO or managed care company. The patient's out-of-pocket expense paid directly to the provider is usually either a fixed dollar amount or percentage of the service cost.

Diagnosis Related Groups (DRGs):   DRGs describe categories of illnesses that might be treated within a certain time frame. DRGs meant that Medicare and Medicaid reimbursement would be based on the diagnosis of the patient instead of the previous formula of cost plus profit.

Empirically Validated Treatments (EVTs):   Specific counseling approaches that have been shown through research to produce effective outcomes for particular client problems.

Employee Retirement Income Securities Act (ERISA, 1974):   Federal legislation designed to protect workers' retirement plans. However, one effect of ERISA is the prevention of any (a) legal action being brought against and (b) government regulations being imposed upon a company that contracts to provide benefits in the workplace.

Fee-for-service: A form of financial reimbursement to the provider based on a set rate for each service rendered; the client selected the provider and received treatment without the insurer's prior approval; the traditional way of paying for treatment before managed care.

Fully insured plans: These are plans where an employer pays for an insurance policy to cover employees' health care. Contrast with self-insured plans.

Gag clauses: Portions of a contract that prevent the therapist from discussing with the client treatment possibilities not covered by the insurance plan.

Gatekeeper: Usually the primary care provider or HMO representative (accessed by phone). A person who first assesses the patient's needs and determines if care from a specialist, a higher costing provider, is necessary. If the gatekeeper is a PCP, he or she often provides care of the illness rather than sending the patient to another provider.

Global Assessment of Functioning (GAF): A scale designed to provide a universal system for clinicians to rank a patient's composite social, occupational, and psychological functioning from a low of zero to a high of 100.

Health Care Finance Agency (HCFA): The federal agency that oversees all health financing policies for Medicare and the Office of Prepaid Health Care. Decisions made by HCFA often result in similar actions by managed care agencies regarding the standard financial worth of each type of service.

Health Maintenance Organization (HMO): A type of managed care system. Any group that provides third-party payment to a provider for services rendered to a voluntarily enrolled prescriber.

Health Plan Employer Data and Information Set (HEDIS): Group of standard measures designed to evaluate health plans.

HMO Act of 1973: Federal legislation that provided $325 million over a five-year period to encourage the startup of new HMOs and the slowing of health care costs. The 1973 HMO act also allowed profit-oriented corporations to become involved in HMOs.

Hold harmless provision: Many managed care or health maintenance organizations have providers sign this clause in their contract indicating that the managed care organization will not be held liable for services rendered by the provider.

Idiographic assessment: Measurements where the focus of attention are elements relatively specific to a particular individual. A depressed person, for example, may exhibit that depression in a unique way. Proposed as a potentially more precise measure of outcome.

Indemnity insurance: Fee-for-service insurance that allows clients to select providers and obtain treatment without the prior approval of the insurer.

Individual or Independent Practice Association (IPA): Major HMOs contract with IPAs to provide services to their members on a capitated basis. IPAs then contract with practitioners or groups of practitioners who are reimbursed on either a fee-for-service or capitated basis.

Informed consent: Mental health providers obtain consent to provide therapy or perform other related procedures from their patients. Informed consent entails that the patient has adequate mental capacity to provide consent, has obtained sufficient knowledge about the procedure(s), has not experienced any coercion or pressure, either direct or indirect, during the decision-making process, and has documented the decision.

Like-provider provision: State statutes may include this requirement for persons on utilization review panels to be health care providers who are specifically trained and licensed in the health care area for which they review services rendered.

Managed Care Organizations (MCO):   The oversight of medical or mental health care delivery by a third-party whose purpose is to limit the care to that which is deemed medically necessary.

Medical necessity: The threshold or standard determination needed for services to be reimbursed by managed care systems. These services are required for or deemed necessary and appropriate for the diagnosis and treatment of medical conditions.

Medical loss ratios: How much money a managed care company spends on health care compared to their profits.

Medical offset effects: Instance where the provision of mental health services can lead to reduced use of medical services. For example, treating clients' depression may lead to fewer visits to the emergency room and to general practitioners.

Medical Savings Accounts (MSAs):   Individuals make tax-free deposits and withdraw money without penalty from these accounts to pay medical expenses or health insurance premiums.

Mental health benefits: Designated and delineated by the managed care system, those services for which the consumer can/will receive reimbursement.

National Committee for Quality Assurance (NCQA):   A private, nonprofit group predominantly composed of representatives from managed care companies and employers designed to evaluate the quality of managed care plans. NCQA accredits managed care organizations on the basis of a standardized review; they began accrediting MCOs in 1991. Also see Health Plan Employer Data and Information Set (HEDIS).

No-cause panel termination: A managed care company's removal of a provider from its panel without showing justification.

Outcome assessment: A method designed to gauge the client's level of progress in therapy. Examples include the GAF and OQ-45.

Patient Bill of Rights: A 1998 piece of federal legislation designed to improve health care through such actions as allowing individuals to see specialists outside of their MC plan at no extra cost and providing children access to pediatric specialists.

"Per thousand" statistic: Often referred to during evaluations of days of inpatient use. Equals number of incidents (e.g., admits, visits) occurring in one month divided by total enrollment times 1,000 or 12,000 for annualized statistics; for example, $N/E \times 12{,}000$. This allows comparison of utilized services across time periods.

Preferred Provider Organization (PPO):   A type of managed care system in which the clients are given financial incentive or required to utilize a specific set of providers (i.e., those formally approved by the company) versus another provider of the clients' choice.

Provider: The health care professional delivering services to members of a managed care company.

Provider panel: The managed care company's list of acceptable providers (i.e., the list of providers who have contracted to provide services to a managed care company's members).

Quality assurance: The establishment of standards of care and the periodic assessment of the appropriateness of those standards.

Self-insured plans: When an employer pays directly for employees' health care. Contrast with fully insured plans.

Short-term therapy: Often referred to as brief psychotherapy, counseling that consists of 8 to 12 sessions.

Third-party payers: An organization or company responsible for paying providers for services rendered to persons who have contracted with the organization for the management of their health care services. Rather than paying directly for services provided, members pay the organization a fixed amount of money in exchange for guaranteed amounts and types of services.

Utilization review: The review of clinical information to determine the medical necessity and appropriateness of services and ensure their cost-effective provision.

Very short-term therapy: Two to four sessions, often the result of HMO's limitations to services.

***Wickline v. State of California* (1987):**   Court case which made it the provider's responsibility to push insurance companies for adequate care. In this case, which involved physical rather than mental health care liability in managed care contexts, the court's decision set the principle for imposing liability on the treating physician for not protesting aggressively the third-party payor's limitations to patient care when those limitations impose upon the physician's medical judgment.

Yellow-dog contracts: Labor agreements designed for and by employers with the main or sole purpose of meeting the employers' needs. The needs of the employees are ignored.

References

Ad Hoc Committee to Defend Health Care. (1997). For our patients, not for profits: A call for action. *Journal of the American Medical Association, 278,* 1733–1739.

Adams, J. F., Piercy, F. P., & Jurich, J. A. (1991). Effects of solution focused therapy's "Formula First Session Task" on compliance and outcome in family therapy. *Journal of Marital & Family Therapy, 17,* 277–290.

Allen, M. G. (1996). Understanding and coping with managed care. In J. Barron and H. Sands (Eds.), *Impact of managed care on psychodynamic treatment* (pp. 15–25). Madison, CT: International Universities Press.

American Psychiatric Association. (1994). *Diagnostic and statistical manual of mental disorders* (4th ed.). Washington, DC: Author.

American Psychological Association. (1992). *Directory of the American Psychological Association: Ethical principles of psychologists.* Washington, DC: Author.

American Psychological Association. (1998). *Interprofessional health care services in primary care settings: Implications for the education and training of psychologists.* Washington, DC: Author.

American Psychological Association. (1999). Bipartisan House proposal includes health plan liability. *Practitioner Update, 7 (2),* 1.

American Rehabilitation Counseling Association. (1987). *Code of professional ethics for rehabilitation counselors.* Arlington Heights, IL: Author.

American School Counselor Association. (1992). *Ethical standards for school counselors.* Alexandria, VA: Author.

Anderson, D. F., Berlant, J. L., Mauch, D., & Maloney, W. (1997). Managed behavioral health care services. In P. Kongstvedt (Ed.), *Essentials of managed health care* (2nd ed.; pp. 248–273). Gaithersburg, MD: Aspen Publications.

Andrews, C. (1995). *Profit fever: The drive to corporatize health care and how to stop it.* Monroe, ME: Common Courage Press.

Association for Specialists in Group Work. (1989). *Ethical guidelines for group counselors.* Alexandria, VA: American Counseling Association.

Auletta, K. (1999, July 26). What I did at summer camp: A reporter gets inside Herb Allen's C.E.O. retreat. *The New Yorker, 75,* 46–51.

Austad, C. (1996). *Is long-term therapy unethical?* San Francisco: Jossey-Bass.

Barber, J. P. (1994). Efficacy of short-term dynamic psychotherapy: Past, present, and future. *Journal of Psychotherapy Practice & Research, 3,* 108–121.

Basco, M. R., Krebaum, S. R., & Rush, A. J. (1997). Outcome measures of depression. In H. H. Strupp, L. M. Horowitz, & M. J. Lambert (Eds.), *Measuring patient changes in mood, anxiety, and personality disorders* (pp. 191–246). Washington, DC: American Psychological Association.

Beisecker, A. E. (1996). Older persons' medical encounters and their outcomes. *Research on Aging, 18,* 9–31.

Bergin, A. E., & Garfield, S. L. (Eds.) (1994). *Handbook of psychotherapy and behavior change* (4th ed.). New York, NY: Wiley.

Bickman, L., & Dokecki, P. (1989). Public and private responsibility for mental health services. *American Psychologist, 44,* 1138–1141.

Birenbaum, A., & Cohen, H. J. (1998). Managed care and quality health services for people with developmental disabilities: Is there a future for UAPs? *Mental Retardation, 36,* 325–329.

Blackwell, B., Gutmann, M., & Gutmann, L. (1988). Case review and quantity of outpatient care. *American Journal of Psychiatry, 145,* 1003–1006.

Brooks, D., & Riley, P. (1998). The impact of managed health care policy on student field training. In G. Schamess & A. Lightburn (Eds.), *Humane managed care?* (pp. 455–464). Washington, DC: NASW Press.

Broskowski, A. (1994). Current mental health care environments: Why managed care is necessary. In R. Lowman & R. Resnick (Eds.), *The mental health professional's guide to managed care* (pp. 1–18). Washington, DC: American Psychological Association.

Brown, J. (1991). *The quality management professional's study guide.* Pasadena, CA: Managed Care Consultants.

Buchholz, S. (1998). The dilemma of managed care. *American Psychologist, 53,* 484–490.

Budman, S. H. (Ed.) (1983). *Forms of brief therapy.* New York: Guilford.

Budman, S. H., & Gurman, A. S. (1996). Theory and practice of brief therapy. In J. E. Groves (Ed.), *Essential papers on short-term dynamic therapy. Essential papers in psychoanalysis* (pp. 43–65). New York, NY: New York University Press.

Burlingame, G. M., Lambert, M. J., Reisinger, C. W., Neff, W. L., & Mosier, J. (1995). Pragmatics of tracking mental health outcomes in a managed care setting. *Journal of Mental Health Administration, 22,* 226–236.

Califano, J. A., Jr. (1986). *America's health care revolution: Who lives? Who dies? Who pays?* New York: Random House.

Canadian Psychological Association. (1991). *Canadian code of ethics for psychologists. Revised.* Ottawa, ON: Author.

Center for Health Economics Research, Brandeis University. (1993). *Access to health care: Key indicators for policy.* Princeton, NJ: Robert Wood Johnson Foundation.

Clement, P. W. (1999). *Outcomes and incomes.* New York: Guilford.

Collins, L. M. (1991). Measurement in longitudinal research. In L. M. Collins & J. L. Horn, *Best methods for the analysis of change* (pp. 137–148). Washington, DC: American Psychological Association.

Committee for the Advancement of Professional Practice. (1995). *CAPP practitioner survey results.* Washington, DC: American Psychological Association.

Constantine, M. G., & Gloria, A. M. (1998). The impact of managed care on predoctoral internship sites: A national survey. *Professional Psychology: Research and Practice, 29,* 195–199.

Corcoran, K., & Vandiver, V. (1996). *Maneuvering the maze of managed care.* New York: Free Press.

Cummings, N. A. (1996). Does managed mental health care offset costs related to medical treatment? In A. Lazarus (Ed.), *Controversies in managed mental health care* (pp. 213–227). Washington, DC: American Psychiatric Press.

Cummings, N., Budman, S., & Thomas, J. (1998). Efficient psychotherapy as a viable response to scarce resources and rationing of treatment. *Professional Psychology: Research & Practice, 29,* 460–469.

Cummings, N., & Sayama, M. (1995). *Focused psychotherapy: A casebook of brief, intermittent psychotherapy throughout the life cycle.* New York: Brunner/Mazel.

Cypres, A., Landsberg, G., & Spellmann, M. (1997). The impact of managed care on community mental health outpatient services in New York state. *Administration & Policy in Mental Health, 24,* 509–521.

Daniels, N., Light, D. W., & Caplan, R. L. (1996). *Benchmarks of fairness for health care reform.* New York: Oxford University Press.

Davidson, K. (1998). Educating students for social work in health care today. In G. Schamess & A. Lightburn (Eds.), *Humane managed care?* (pp. 425–429). Washington, DC: NASW Press.

Davis, K. (1998). Managed health care: Forcing social work to make choices and changes. In G. Schamess & A. Lightburn (Eds.), *Humane managed care?* (pp. 409–429). Washington, DC: NASW Press.

Dean, J., & Feder, J. (1999). Union affiliation update. *NYSPA Notebook, 11,* 7.

DeLeon, P. H., VandenBos, G. R., & Bulatao, E. Q. (1994). Managed mental health care: A history of the federal policy initiative. In R. Lowman & R. Resnick (Eds.), *The mental health professional's guide to managed care* (pp. 19–40). Washington, DC: American Psychological Association.

Di Palo, M. T. (1997). Rating satisfaction research: Is it __Poor, __Fair, __Good, __ Very Good, or __Excellent? *Arthritic Care & Research, 10,* 422–430.

Does therapy help? (1995, November). *Consumer Reports, 60,* 734–739.

Donner, S. (1998). Fieldwork crisis: Dilemmas, dangers, and opportunities. In G. Schamess & A. Lightburn (Eds.), *Humane managed care?* (pp. 442–454). Washington, DC: NASW Press.

Endicott, J., Spitzer, R., Fleiss, J., & Cohen, J. (1976). The Global Assessment Scale: A procedure for measuring overall severity of psychiatric disturbance. *Archives of General Psychiatry, 33,* 766–771.

Epstein, E. E., McCrady, B. S., Miller, K. J., & Steinberg, M. (1994). Attrition from conjoint alcoholism treatment: Do dropouts differ from completers? *Journal of Substance Abuse, 6,* 249–265.

Finkelstein, K. E. (1997). The sick business: Why for-profit medicine couldn't care less. *The New Republic, 217,* 23.

Fox, P. D. (1997). An overview of managed care. In P. Kongstvedt (Ed.), *Essentials of managed health care* (2nd ed.; pp. 3–16). Gaithersburg, MD: Aspen Publications.

Frank, J. (1971). Therapeutic factors in psychotherapy. *American Journal of Psychotherapy, 25,* 350–361.

Galewitz, P. (1999a, July 14). Study says for-profit HMOs provide inferior care. *Buffalo News,* A1.

Galewitz, P. (1999b, November 12). New HMO policy excludes mental health care. *Buffalo News,* A14.

Gaston, L., & Sabourin, S. (1992). Client satisfaction and social desirability in psychotherapy. *Evaluation and Program Planning, 15,* 227–231.

Giles, T. R. (1993). *Managed mental health care.* Allyn and Bacon: Boston.

Glasser, R. J. (1998). The doctor is not in: On the managed failure of managed health care. *Harper's Magazine, 296,* 35.

Goldberg, C. (January 23, 2000). For many states, health care bills are top priority. *New York Times,* 1–18.

Goodman, M., Brown, J., & Deitz, P. (1992). *Managing managed care: A mental health practitioner's survival guide.* Washington, DC: American Psychiatric Press. [case histories start on p. 44]

Gottlieb, G. L. (1995). The changing marketplace for mental health services: The challenge for freestanding psychiatry. *Psychiatric Annals, 25,* 500–503.

Gray, B. (1991). *The profit motive and patient care.* Cambridge, MA: Harvard University Press.

Gronlund, N. E. (1988). *Measurement and evaluation in teaching* (5th ed.). New York: Macmillan.

Grossberg, S. H. (1997). The mechanics of developing a successful behavioral group practice for managed care: How to survive in the competitive field of mental health practice. In R. M. Alperin & D. G. Phillips (Eds.), *The impact of managed care on the practice of psychotherapy: Innovation, implementation, and controversy* (pp. 31–40). New York, NY, USA: Brunner/Mazel.

Gunzburger, D., Henggeler, S., & Watson, S. (1985). Factors related to premature termination of counseling relationships. *Journal of College Student Personnel, 26,* 456–460.

Haas, L. J., & Cummings, N. A. (1994). Managed outpatient mental health plans: Clinical, ethical, and practical guidelines for participation. In R. Lowman & R. Resnick (Eds.), *The mental health professional's guide to managed care* (pp. 137–150). Washington, DC: American Psychological Association.

Hayes, S., Nelson, R., & Jarrett, R. (1987). The treatment utility of assessment: A functional approach to evaluating assessment quality. *American Psychologist, 42,* 963–974.

Haynes, K., & Mickelson, J. (2000). *Affecting change : Social workers in the political arena* (4th ed.). New York: Allyn & Bacon.

Hayslip, B., Hoffman, J., & Weatherly, D. (1990–1991). Response bias in hospice evaluation. *Omega, 22,* 63–74.

Herlihy, B., & Corey, G. (Eds.) (1996). *ACA ethical standards casebook* (5th ed.). Alexandria, VA: American Counseling Association.

Herndon, J. E., Fleishman, S., Kosty, M. P., & Green, M. R. (1997). A longitudinal study of quality of life in advanced non-small cell lung cancer: Cancer and Leukemia Group B (CALGB) 8931. *Controlled Clinical Trials, 13,* 286–300.

Higuchi, S. (1994). Recent managed-care legislative and legal issues. In R. Lowman & R. Resnick (Eds.), *The mental health professional's guide to managed care* (pp. 83–118). Washington, DC: American Psychological Association.

Hill, C. E., & O'Brien, K. M. (1999). *Helping skills.* Washington, DC: American Psychological Association.

Himmelstein, D., Woolhandler, S., Hellander, I., & Wolfe, S. (1999). Quality of care in investor-owned vs not-for-profit HMOs. *Journal of the American Medical Association, 282,* 159–63.

Howard, K., Kopta, S., Krause, M., & Orlinsky, D. (1986). The dose-effect relationship in psychotherapy. *American Psychologist, 41,* 159–164.

Hurley, R. E., Kirschner, L., & Bone, T. W. (1997). Medicaid managed care. In P. Kongstvedt (Ed.), *Essentials of managed health care* (2nd ed.; pp. 432–450). Gaithersburg, MD: Aspen Publications.

Iglehart, J. K. (1996). Managed care and mental health. *Health Policy Report, 334,* 131–135.

Jackson, M. (April 11, 1999). CEOs too cozy with compensation committees? *Buffalo News,* A3.

Jost, K. (1998). Managed care and its discontents. *Congressional Quarterly Weekly Report, 56,* S5.

Kadera, S. W., Lambert, M. J., & Andrews, A. A. (1996). How much therapy is really enough? *Journal of Psychotherapy Practice and Research, 5,* 132–151.

Kassan, L. D. (1996). *Shrink rap: Sixty psychotherapists discuss their work, their lives, and the state of their field.* Northvale, NJ: Aronson.

Kazdin, A. E. (1996). Dropping out of child psychotherapy: Issues for research and implications for practice. *Clinical Child Psychology and Psychiatry, 1,* 133–156.

Kessler, K. A. (1998). History of managed behavioral health care and speculations about its future. *Harvard Review of Psychiatry, 6,* 155–159.

Kiesler, C. A., Cummings, N. A., & VandenBos, G. R. (Eds.) (1979). *Psychology and national health insurance: A sourcebook.* Washington, DC: American Psychological Association.

Kongstvedt, P. (1997). Common operational problems in managed health care plans. In P. Kongstvedt (Ed.), *Essentials of managed health care* (2nd ed.; pp. 391–402). Gaithersburg, MD: Aspen Publications.

Kopta, S. M., Howard, K. I., Lowry, J. L., & Beutler, L. E. (1994). Patterns of symptomatic recovery in psychotherapy. *Journal of Consulting & Clinical Psychology, 62,* 1009–1016.

Kuttner, R. (1999). Wall Street and health care: The American health care system. *New England Journal of Medicine, 340,* 664–669.

Lambert, M. J., & Hill, C. E. (1994). Assessing psychotherapy outcomes and processes. In A. E. Bergin & S. L. Garfield (Eds.), *Handbook of psychotherapy & behavior change* (pp. 72–113). New York: Wiley.

Lambert, M. J., & Huefner, J. C. (1996, August 9). *Measuring outcomes in clinical practice.* Workshop conducted at the Annual Meeting of the American Psychological Association, Toronto.

LeBow, J. L. (1983). Client satisfaction with mental health treatment. *Evaluation Review, 7,* 729–752.

Leff, H. S., & Woocher, L. S. (1997). Trends in the evaluation of managed mental health care. In G. Schamess & A. Lightburn (Eds.), *Humane managed care?* (pp. 477–481). Washington, DC: NASW Press.

Lewis, J. R. (1994). Patient views on quality care in general practice: Literature review. *Social Science & Medicine, 39,* 655–670.

Lieberman, T. (1999). How does your HMO stack up? *Consumer Reports,* August, 1999.

Lopez, F. G. (1985). Brief therapy: A model for early counselor training. *Counselor Education & Supervision, 24,* 307–316.

Lowman, R. (1994). Mental health claims experience: Analysis and benefit redesign. In R. Lowman & R. Resnick (Eds.), *The mental health professional's guide to managed care* (pp. 119–136). Washington, DC: American Psychological Association.

Lowman, R., & Resnick, R. (Eds.) (1994). *The mental health professional's guide to managed care.* Washington, DC: American Psychological Association.

Lubin, H., Loris, M., Burt, J., & Johnson, D. (1998). Efficacy of psychoeducational group therapy in reducing symptoms of posttraumatic stress disorder among multiply traumatized women. *American Journal of Psychiatry, 155,* 1172–1177.

Magellan Behavioral Health. (1999). A closer look at NCQA. *Provider Focus, 2,* 4–5.

Major, W. (1999, August). Quality Management Program works to improve health care in the community. *Independent Health Scope, 2,* 1–4.

McGuire, P. (1998). Kaiser therapists stage one-day strike. *APA Monitor, 39,* 22.

Mechanic, D. (1997). The future of inpatient psychiatry in general hospitals. In D. Mechanic (Ed.), *Improving inpatient psychiatric treatment in an era of managed care* (pp. 103–108). San Francisco, CA: Jossey-Bass.

Meckler, L. (April 27, 1999). Senate debates cost of Democratic HMO bill. *Buffalo News,* A6.

Meier, S. (1994). *The chronic crisis in psychological measurement and assessment.* New York: Academic Press.

Meier, S. (1997). Nomothetic item selection rules for tests of psychological interventions. *Psychotherapy Research, 7,* 419–427.

Meier, S. (1998). Evaluating change-based item selection rules. *Measurement and Evaluation in Counseling and Development, 31,* 15–27.

Meier, S. T. (1999). Training the practitioner-scientist: Bridging case conceptualization, assessment, and intervention. *The Counseling Psychologist, 27,* 846–869.

Meier, S. T., & Davis, S. R. (1990). Trends in reporting psychometric properties of instruments employed in counseling psychology research. *Journal of Counseling Psychology, 37,* 113–115.

Meier, S. T., & Davis, S. R. (2000). *The elements of counseling* (4th ed.). Pacific Grove, CA: Brooks/Cole.

Meier, S. T., & Letsch, E. (in press). What is necessary and sufficient information for outcome assessment? *Professional Psychology: Research & Practice.*

Meyer, G. J., Finn, S. E., Eyde, L. D., Kay, G. G., Kubiszy, T. W., Moreland, K. L., Eisman, E. J., & Dies, R. R. (1998). *Benefits and costs of psychological assessment in healthcare delivery: Report of the Board of Professional Affairs Psychological Assessment Work Group, Part I.* Washington, DC: American Psychological Association.

Miller, I. J. (1995). Managed care is harmful to outpatient mental health services: A call for accountability. *Professional Psychology: Research and Practice, 27,* 349–363.

Miller, I. J. (1996). Ethical and liability issues concerning invisible rationing. *Professional Psychology: Research and Practice, 27,* 583–587.

Miller, J. (1998). Managed care and merger mania: Strategies for preserving clinical social work education. In G. Schamess & A. Lightburn (Eds.), *Humane managed care?* (pp. 465–476). Washington, DC: NASW Press.

Moldawsky, S. (1990). Is solo practice really dead? *American Psychologist, 45,* 544–546.

Mordock, J. B. (1996). The road to survival revisited: Organizational adaptation to the managed care environment. *Child Welfare, LXXV,* 195–218.

Morse, D. (1998). Confronting existential anxiety: The ultimate stressor. *Stress Medicine, 14,* 109–119.

Mueller, R. M., Lambert, M. J., & Burlingame, G. M. (1998). Construct validity of the Outcome Questionnaire: A confirmatory factor analysis. *Journal of Personality Assessment, 70,* 248–262.

National Association of School Psychologists. (1992). *Principles for professional ethics.* Silver Spring, MD: Author.

National Association of Social Workers. (1994). *NASW code of ethics.* Washington, DC: Author.

National Board for Certified Counselors. (1989). *National Board for Certified Counselors: Code of Ethics.* Alexandria, VA: Author.

National Career Development Association. (1987). *National Career Development Association ethical standards.* Alexandria, VA: Author.

Newman, R., & Bricklin, P. M. (1994). Parameters of managed mental health care: Legal, ethical, and professional guidelines. In R. Lowman & R. Resnick (Eds.), *The mental health professional's guide to managed care* (pp. 63–82). Washington, DC: American Psychological Association.

Newman, R., & Reed, G. M. (1996). Psychology as a health care profession: Its evolution and future directions. In R. J. Resnick & R. H. Rozensky (Eds.), *Health psychology through the life span: Practice and research opportunities* (pp. 11–26). Washington, DC: American Psychological Association.

Norton, M. C., Breitner, J. C. S., Welsh, K. A., & Wyse, B. W. (1994). Characteristics of nonresponders in a community survey of the elderly. *Journal of the American Geriatrics Society, 42,* 1252–1256.

Odell, M., & Quinn, W. H. (1998). Therapist and client behaviors in the first interview: Effects on session impact and treatment duration. *Journal of Marriage & Family Counseling, 24,* 369–388.

Ogles, B. M., Lambert, M. J., & Masters, K. S. (1996). *Assessing outcome in clinical practice.* New York: Allyn & Bacon.

Parvin, R., & Anderson, G. (1995). Monetary issues. In E. J. Rave & C. C. Larsen (Eds.), *Ethical decision making in therapy: Feminist perspectives* (pp. 57–87). New York, NY: Guilford Press.

Patterson, D., & Sharfstein, S. (1992). The future of mental health care. In J. Feldman & R. Fitzpatrick (Eds.), *Managed mental health care: Administration and clinical issues* (pp. 335–343). Washington, DC: American Psychiatric Press.

Pedulla, D. M., & Rocke, S. (1999). Demystifying ERISA: Understanding the basics of a complex law. *APA Practitioner Focus, 12,* 2–18.

Pikoff, H. (1996). *Treatment effectiveness handbook.* Buffalo, NY: Data for Decisions.

Rabasca, L. (1999). Health plans continue to limit mental health benefits, study finds. *APA Monitor, 30,* 10.

Richardson, L. M., & Austad, C. S. (1994). Realities of mental health practices in managed-care settings. In R. Lowman & R. Resnick (Eds.), *The mental health professional's guide to managed care* (pp. 151–168). Washington, DC: American Psychological Association.

Roback, H. B., & Smith, M. (1987). Patient attrition in dynamically oriented treatment groups. *American Journal of Psychiatry, 144,* 426–431.

Roberts, A. R. (1998). Inhumane versus humane managed care. In G. Schamess & A. Lightburn (Eds.), *Humane managed care?* (pp. 505–507). Washington, DC: NASW Press.

Rochefort, D. A. (1997). *From poorhouses to homelessness: Policy analysis and mental health care* (2nd ed.). Westport, CT: Auburn House/Greenwood Publishing.

Sands, H., Cullen, E., & Higuchi, S. (1996). Practitioner's alert: Health care fraud and abuse. *Psychoanalysis & Psychotherapy, 13,* 86–88.

Sauber, S. R. (Ed.) (1997a). *Managed mental health care.* Bristol, PA: Brunner/Mazel.

Sauber, S. R. (1997b). Introduction to managed mental health care: Provider survival. In S. R. Sauber (Ed.), *Managed mental health care* (pp. 1–39). Bristol, PA: Brunner/Mazel.

Schamess, G., & Lightburn, A. (Eds.) (1998). *Humane managed care?* Washington, DC: NASW Press.

Scheffler, R., & Ivey, S. L. (1998). Mental health staffing in managed care organizations: A case study. *Psychiatric Services, 49,* 1303–1308.

Sexton, T. L., Whiston, S. C., Bleuer, J. C., & Walz, G. R. (1997). *Integrating outcome research into counseling practice and training.* Alexandria, Va: American Counseling Association.

Shore, K. (1996). Beyond managed care and managed competition. *The Independent Practitioner: Bulletin of the Division of Independent Practice, Division 42 of the American Psychological Association, 16,* 24–25.

Silverman, C., & Miller, S. I. (1994). Drugs and alcohol: The managed care view. In R. K. Schreter & S. S. Sharfstein (Eds.), *Allies and adversaries: The impact of managed care on mental health services* (pp. 85–99). Washington, DC: American Psychiatric Press.

Sitzia, J., & Wood, N. (1997). Patient satisfaction: A review of issues and concepts. *Social Science & Medicine, 45,* 1829–1843.

Smith, M. L., Glass, G. V., & Miller, T. I. (1980). *The benefits of psychotherapy.* Baltimore: The Johns Hopkins Press.

Sommers-Flanagan, R., & Sommers-Flanagan, J. (1999). *Clinical interviewing* (2nd ed.). New York, NY: John Wiley & Sons.

Speer, D. C., & Newman, F. L. (1996). Mental health services outcome evaluation. *Clinical Psychology: Science & Practice, 3,* 105–129.

Speer, D. C., & Zold, A. C. (1971). An example of self-selection bias in follow-up research. *Journal of Clinical Psychology, 27,* 64–68.

Spiggle, D. L., & Hughes, D. H. (1998). Is managed care managing not to care? *Psychiatric Services, 49,* 1545–1546.

Spitzer, R. L., Gibbon, M., Williams, J. B. W., & Endicott, J. (1996). Global Assessment of Functioning (GAF) Scale. In L. I. Sederer & B. Dickey (Eds.), *Outcomes assessment in clinical practice* (pp. 76–78). Baltimore, MD: Williams & Wilkins.

Stallard, P. (1996). The role and use of consumer satisfaction surveys in mental health services. *Journal of Mental Health, 5,* 333–348.

Stark, M. J. (1992). Dropping out of substance abuse treatment: A clinically oriented review. *Clinical Psychology Review, 12,* 93–116.

Steenbarger, B. N. (1994). Duration and outcome in psychotherapy: An integrative review. *Professional Psychology: Research and Practice, 25,* 111–119.

Strupp, H. H., Horowitz, L. M., & Lambert, M. J. (1997). *Measuring patient changes in mood, anxiety, and personality disorders.* Washington, DC: American Psychological Association.

Sue, S. (1999). Science, ethnicity, and bias. *American Psychologist, 54,* 1070–1077.

Sykes-Wylie, M. (1994). Endangered species. *Family Therapy Networker, 18,* 20–33.

Tryon, W. W. (1991). *Activity measurement in psychology and medicine.* New York: Plenum.

Vandivort-Warren, R. (1998). How social workers can manage managed care. In G. Schamess & A. Lightburn (Eds.), *Humane managed care?* (pp. 255–267). Washington, DC: NASW Press.

VanLeit, B. (1996). Managed mental health care: Reflections in a time of turmoil. *The American Journal of Occupational Therapy, 50,* 428–434.

Weisz, J., Huey, S., & Weersing, V. (1998). Psychotherapy outcome research with children and adolescents. In T. Ollendick & R. Prinz (Eds.), *Advances in clinical child psychology* (Vol. 20; pp. 49–91). New York: Plenum.

Weinstock, M. C. (1999). *Measuring change in university counseling center clients.* Unpublished dissertation, SUNY Buffalo.

Welch, B. L. (1999). Psychoanalysis in the political arena: The reality principle. In H. Kaley, M. Eagle, & D. Wolitzky (Eds.), *Psychoanalytic therapy as health care: Effectiveness and economics in the 21st century* (pp. 3–13). Hillsdale, NJ: The Analytic Press.

Welfel, E. (1998). *Ethics in counseling and psychotherapy: Standards, research, and emerging issues.* Pacific Grove, CA: Wadsworth.

Wierzbicki, M., & Pekarik, G. (1993). A meta-analysis of psychotherapy dropout. *Professional Psychology: Research and Practice, 24,* 190–195.

Wiger, D. (1999). *The clinical documentation sourcebook: A comprehensive collection of mental health practice forms, handouts, and records* (2nd ed.). New York: Wiley.

Yenney, S. L. (1994). *Business strategies for a caring profession.* Washington, DC: American Psychological Association.

Zarabozo, C., & LeMasurier, J. D. (1997). Medicare and managed care. In P. Kongstvedt (Ed.), *Essentials of managed health care* (2nd ed.; pp. 405–431). Gaithersburg, MD: Aspen Publications.

Zinbarg, R., Craske, M., & Barlow, D. (1993). *Therapist's guide for the mastery of your anxiety and worry.* Albany, NY: Graywind Publications Incorporated.

Index